Essays on Acupuncture

Michael Keane, D.Ac.

Michael Keane Creative Studios

Publishing Information

Michael Keane Creative Studios:

If you would like to support our efforts, consider visiting *Herb and Needle*, an educational content hub for acupuncture and herbal medicine. Our website is www.herbandneedle.com. Our goal is the continued production of educational content, works, creations, books and other resources for the goal of making acupuncture and herbal medicine more understandable, fun, and grounded in tradition and science — and to transmit this out to the world.

This project is a part of Michael Keane Creative Studios. We are an independent, individually run project at the junction of art and science.

With profound gratitude,

Michael Keane

Author Information:

Michael Keane, D.Ac. is an acupuncturist and herbalist with over a decade of experience currently practicing in Salt Lake City, Utah at a high-volume clinic downtown called SLC Qi, as well as a multidisciplinary artist, painter, author, and creator. He teaches graduate students at the Won Institute of Graduate Studies and creates educational content and materials for acupuncture and herbal medicine through his brand, *Herb and Needle*.

His personal artwork can be found on his website: www.michaelkeane.art.

This book is dedicated to all of my mentors, teachers, and patients who have been a part of my journey in the healing arts throughout the years.

A special thanks go out to Matt Jevtic and the entire SLC Qi crew.

Preface

I started writing this book with the literary essays of Emerson in mind, as well as the styles of writing found in the *Analects of Confucius*, *Dao De Jing*, and other ancient Chinese philosophical texts which I explore, revisit and study. I was particularly influenced by my readings of the *Nei Jing Su Wen* and *Ling Shu*. These are perhaps the two most fundamental texts of Classical Chinese Medicine. Their quotes are littered throughout the essays as I felt compelled to interweave them throughout—they were so fresh on my mind and my practice at the time of writing parts of this book. I found that it made the writing process more interesting for me and it created a comparative philosophy dynamic between my own ideas, language, and the classical quotes. The writing of this book also coincided with a long ongoing translation project of mine of the *Zhenjiu Dacheng*, so this magnificent acupuncture text also featured prominently in the quotations and in my world experience at the time.

The essays are not intended to be in any particular order, similar to how the *Analects of Confucius* are presented, although I did strive to group similar topics within proximity to one another for the convenience of the reader. The one piece of major structural organization of the book takes place in the division of the materials into three different sections.

Essays on Acupuncture

1. **Needling Techniques**, which includes essays on practical techniques for using needles in the clinic.

2. **External Essays**, which include topics about how to do acupuncture, such as theory, practice, and general concepts, and perspectives on the art, tradition, and science of acupuncture.

3. **Internal Essays**, which include topics which have to do with the condition of an acupuncturist, such as inner disposition, mental emotional or spiritual state, behaviors, and topics important for inner growth.

Contents

"The principles of acupuncture are easy to say but difficult to master."
Ling Shu, Chapter 1

"Those who are experts in the use of the needles, when they remove an illness, that is as if they pulled out a thorn, as if they cleansed a stain, as if they untied a knot, as if they opened a closure. The illness may have lasted for long, and still it can be brought to an end. Those who state that it cannot be cured, they simply have not acquired the necessary skills."
Ling Shu, Chapter 1

"Beware, beware! The perfect Way is subtle! Its changes and transformations are inexhaustible. Who would know its origin? How embarrassing: even exemplary people, they are helpless; who of them knows its essentials? In view of the unfathomable, who can stand up to this?"
Su Wen, Chapter 8

Needling Methods

There are many different needling techniques and each technique serves a different purpose, and accordingly, has advantages or disadvantages. Through study, practice and learning, we apply creative reasoning to choose the appropriate techniques, just as a craftsman utilizes the compass or square to measure and plan, or chooses the right tools for the job at hand. It is not uncommon to employ multiple techniques together in a single treatment to unlock synergistic actions. One must have a deep understanding and command of the foundations of each in order to unlock the possibilities. This comes with continuous study, practice, and learning.

The classic on acupuncture, the *Ling Shu*, discusses the topic of needle techniques in-depth and should be studied closely by every acupuncturist. Essays in this section overview various techniques which might be utilized in practice but it is by no means an exhaustive list of all possibilities.

Triple Needle Acupuncture

Dào Mǎ 道馬

For the large majority of instances it is useful to employ the triple acupuncture needling technique which was innovated and used by Master Tung, which he called *Dao Ma* needling—literally "leading horse," or sometimes rendered as "guiding horse". This is done by selecting a point as the central or main point, and then also needling each adjacent point 1 cun away on both sides.

This needling technique applies a stronger 'dosage' of acupuncture to the zone of the chosen treatment point. Research studies have shown that this method causes powerful De Qi sensations and that it has the most significant effect on modulating neural networks of the brain compared to either a single needle, or a single needle with rotation or thrusting stimulation applied to it.[1]

This method of needling was developed by Master Tung after he concluded that one or two needles were not providing the therapeutic efficacy which he sought. "The Dao Ma System utilizes three needles in different configurations (namely: Three Continuous, Three Transverse, and Three Triangular needles) to address a myriad of disorders and is flexible enough to adapt to virtually any clinical situation."[2]

This is not to say that other methods are inferior or should not be utilized when appropriate. Perhaps in some cases we can even use more than three needles, or only use one if someone is sensitive and it is better to be gentle. Dao Ma is my default method because it is an effective, reliable, and rational approach.

---

1. Effect of acupuncture 'dose' on modulation of the default mode network of the brain.

2. Advanced Tung Style Acupuncture: The Dao Ma Needling Technique of Master Tung Ching-Chang.

Trigger Points

Trigger point needling is a very physical type of needling in the sense that it specifically focuses on releasing muscles, fascial knots and soft tissue adhesions. It can create a strong sensation in the form of tissue fasciculations and it is often quite effective for releasing adhesions and knots, but it may not address the root issue which causes the tension pattern from which the knot arose. One way to improve its efficacy is by combining it with a fuller acupuncture strategy which addresses the Qi and Spirit such as distal points. This allows for treatment of the propensity for the knotting of the Qi (the root) as well as the branch (the knot itself).

For stubborn muscles where one can feel a stagnant knot, such as a palpable nodule in the muscle from which the pain is referred, this type of treatment can be employed. Isolate the knot, fascial adhesion, or nodule with the off-hand and direct the needle into the belly of the knot with the needling hand. The off-hand is just as important as the needling hand for needling accuracy.

> *"Those who understand needling trust in their left [hand]. Those who do not understand needling trust in their right [hand]."*
> *Nan Jing, Chapter 78*

Sometimes this immediately creates a strong Qi fasciculation, releasing the knot. It is important to feel these reactions with the hand in order to be aware of what is happening. At times, we may have to use a firm but gentle thrusting technique to get the Qi to move and react. Faster is not better; it should be a gentle, moderate, firm, deliberate tempo, with extra caution and awareness of fragile structures and organs which may lie underneath.

Even if the knot is released, it must be understood that the condition will often not permanently resolve at the root with this technique and it may eventually return. The patient very likely will go back to the very life processes and habits which caused the propensity for the knot to form. The acupuncturist must use other methods to also treat the deeper root patterns of Qi which are causing this issue, as well as communication to advise the patient on lifestyle changes to alter their causative habits.

This technique takes practice in order to master and perform effectively and safely. There are some areas on the body where it is dangerous to perform if the practitioner is inexperienced, such as the chest, near the clavicle, neck and upper back. Areas near fragile structures or above vulnerable organs like the Lungs require extreme caution. It should not be performed by inexperienced acupuncturists, but unfortunately this is often the most common needling technique that is being taught to them today.

Ashi Points

Ā Shì Xué 阿是穴

Unlike 'normal' acupuncture points, which are specifically designated on the charts and found in the natural crevices of the body where Qi flows along channels, *ashi* points are areas which are tender with palpation. They are non-specific locations where one can observe a palpable change in the tissue such as an emptiness, a stagnation, or some other abnormal tissue manifestation. They also exist as tender points on the channels. Mastering ashi points adds a dimension to our treatments by providing a direct tactile, intuitive element.

There is a saying: "wherever there is pain, there is a point." This quote hints to the practical value of ashi points, which can manifest and be found anywhere on the body. Ashi points can be diagnostic because they can give us information about the nature and root cause of a pain or a pathology. They can also have treatment value, and be used as treatment points depending on the situation. Try mixing local ashi points in with your chosen distal points or palpate to find mirroring holographic areas to find distal ashi points. This is part of Dr. Richard Tan's strategy.

> *"Use the acupuncture points which are painful."*
> *Ling Shu, Chapter 13*

Ashi points often exist on other parts of the body along the channels which holographically mirror the location of pain pathologies. In these cases, they can corroborate a diagnosis as well as be used as points for the treatment of it. Utilize the inherent connections of the Jingluo channels to anticipate where ashi points will lie. The palpated pain associated with them is a resonance which is representative of the disease and Qi pathology. It can be interpreted as a signal from the body to the practitioner that this is an 'active' treatment point.

Preparing the Point

It can be very beneficial to use our hands and palpatory skills to prepare the point which we are going to needle. This is because we aim to always needle gracefully and minimize pain during insertion, which is detrimental to the overall quality and efficacy of the treatment. We simply seek to attain the Qi at the point, not cause a sharp pain at the skin surface during insertion. By using our hands, we can help to smooth and disperse the Qi and blood at the location of the acupuncture point before needling it. This can be done by massaging or stroking the channel which we seek to needle, and by pressing and massaging upon the acupuncture point with our thumb, and even by using our fingernail to push into it somewhat, leaving an indentation. If there is a lot of stagnation at a point, try massaging the point first before needling. Doing this reduces the chances of a painful insertion by dispersing and scattering the Qi and blood at the point. Palpation in general should be somewhat of a reflexive practice, as it also helps us to find the living points that much more accurately.

> *Whenever one inserts the needle, using the left hand thumb's fingernail, firmly press the acupoint being needled to cause the dispersal of Qi and blood. Then afterwards inserting the needle does not injure the nutritive or the defensive [Qi].*
> *Ode of the Twelve-Step Manual Method, from the Zhenjiu Dacheng*

These methods can also be used during and after needle insertion or needle withdrawal. The aim is to smooth the flow of Qi and blood in the channel where it is stagnant or excessive. Massaging the channels and collaterals can guide and circulate the Qi and blood, which can help when it is difficult to attain the Qi. If the patient's Qi is stagnant or blocked, using pressure from our hands and fingers can help to unblock these obstructions. If they exist, they can be clearly felt by the hands when we explore the channel's pathway.

> *Whenever one inserts the needle, if below the needle there is stagnant evil Qi that is rough and unmoving, follow the channel and collateral up and down. Using the thumb's fingernail to press it, their Qì naturally unblocks. The grasping method requires knowledge of the channel Qi stagnation. One must cut with the nail, never too gently.*
> *Ode of the Twelve-Step Manual Method, from the Zhenjiu Dacheng*

Applying dynamic healing touch and palpation methods in this way can be very helpful and aid the acupuncture process immensely. A lot can be accomplished with the hands; we should regard them as our most important clinical tools.

Needling Between Pathways

Sometimes when performing acupuncture it is beneficial to treat multiple channels at once. This can be achieved without employing excessive numbers of needles. Instead of using points on multiple channels we can use acupuncture locations which straddle the location in between two channels, or between two points, to exert influence on multiple areas at the same time. Instead of looking at the channels as a solid line, imagine them as a gradient bleeding into one another at the borderlines.

For example, if we want to treat both the Stomach Foot Yangming and the Gallbladder Foot Shaoyang, we could choose a point which resides between both channels. By finding the midpoint between both channels, an area which lies on the *bordering territory* of both, the point will theoretically have an effect on both channels' related pathways. Certain acupuncture points, such as LU7 or ST40, naturally have this quality by virtue of their positioning. But we can also find our own, non-traditional acupuncture points in these border zones depending upon the context of the situation. Sometimes they appear as ashi points, tender to the touch.

A great example of a point which utilizes this strategy is the Tung acupuncture point *Se San Li* (Beside ST36). This point lies lateral to ST36, closer to the GB channel than the normal ST36 point, but close enough to the original location that it is still resonant with Stomach Yangming. Similarly, we can think of ST40 as a point which naturally resides on the borderlands of both of these channels. Utilize a Dao Ma along this middle-ground to influence both the Yangming and the Shaoyang for a broader effect.

By this logic, a point like *Ce San Li* can be thought of as treating *both* the Earth and Wood phases, and it might be used for disorders involving a disharmony of Wood overacting on Earth, or Wood overcoming the Earth. If a patient has pain which is present on both Yangming and Shaoyang zones, utilizing a point which treats both channels simultaneously may improve the effect. It also means that this point influences the other areas treated by Yangming and Shaoyang, such as the Spleen or the Liver.

Needling Multiple Pathways

It can be advantageous to needle multiple pathways at once. Similar to how one may perform a *Dao Ma* technique down the pathway of a single channel, there are many opportunities to do this in a perpendicular manner, cutting across multiple channels at once. One example of this concept in action would be needling ST36, *Ce San Li*, and GB34.

Using this example to highlight the uses of this strategy, we can see how this channel and point selection method treats a broader range of terrain than if we were to simply choose one channel alone. These three points treat the ST and GB, and *Ce San Li* treats the spaces in between. By applying the systems of mutual channel relationships, these points also reach through to all of the mutual and reciprocal channels of these two pathways. So where a *Dao Ma* on the ST channel alone would be useful for treating ST, SP, LI, and PC, by adding in just the GB channel we also are able to also reach the treatment effects into the LV, SJ, HT and GB. Small modifications and the addition of a single point can turn a unidimensional point selection into a dynamic, multidimensional one.

Pain can exist along multiple channel pathways, so having the flexible option of applying our point selection in novel ways like this gives us treatment options that are less static and more adaptable to practical situations. We may find ourselves in treatment scenarios where the presentation is not clear-cut and the pain or disease exists along multiple channels simultaneously, so we will have to apply our creative reasoning for novel strategic solutions. Life is rarely simplistic, so our treatments must be able to approach the complexities of each manifestation. Master Tung employs this strategy in many of his *Dao Ma* groups, and they are often great examples of this concept in practice. They are all worth studying and deciphering to understand the intentions and the mechanics behind them. We can use this as a theoretical basis to create our own *Dao Ma* point combinations as well.

Other illustrative examples:

Example 1: *Ling Gu* and *Da Bai, Yao Tong Xue*

Example 2: LV3, ST44, GB41

Example 3: SP9, LV7, KD10

Example 4: A horizontal shoulder Dao Ma with LI15 as the central point plus a shoulder point on the Lung channel on one side and SJ14 on the other side.

Example 5: ST36, *Ce San Li*, GB34

Superficial and Deep Needling

Some diseases occur in the exterior, while others exist interiorly. Understanding how to access the different depths of the body with different needle techniques is critical for reaching the correct location and fractal holographic dimension where the illness resides. Accuracy in needling depth will create a more effective treatment.

> *"When the body is first diseased but it has not penetrated to the viscera, the needling should be as half."*
> *Ling Shu, Chapter 6*

The body has different depths, each relating to levels of Yin and Yang. The surface, superficial layers of the body are related to the Yang. This is where the Wei defensive Yang Qi resides. The depths are related to the Yin. This is where the Ying constructive Yin Qi resides. This Yin and Yang relationship extends to pulse diagnosis, acupuncture needling and indeed for the universe as a whole. Depending on where the illness is located one would choose to needle superficially deeply, or in between. This is spoken of in the *Ling Shu*:

> *"The three depths of acupuncture causes the Valley Qi to come out. First it is shallow needling through the skin to let out the Yang evil, then the needling to let out the Yin evil. Whether the Qi is sparse or abundant, go deeply through the skin until reaching the muscles and the flesh. To complete entry into the divisions of the flesh will result in the Valley Qi coming out. Thus, the 'Rule of Acupuncture' says: "To begin, needle shallowly in order to expel the evil Qi and let the Blood and Qi come forward. Afterwards, needle deeply in order to affect the Yin Qi's evil. Finally, needle extremely deeply*

in order to descend to the Valley Qi."
Ling Shu, Chapter 7

Needling depth is also influenced by the seasons based on the microcosm-macrocosm principle. Thus, fluctuations of the seasonal Qi inform our practice. We can remain adaptive and responsive to these subtleties.

Spring and Summer: Shallow Needling During spring and summer, Yang Qi moves upward and floats to the exterior of the body. Because the body's energy is at the Yang surface, pathogenic evils also reside shallowly, meaning that deep needling is not indicated. To correspond with this natural outward expansion, needles must be inserted shallowly or superficially.

- In Spring: The Qi lies within the fine body hair and the superficial connecting vessels located in the partings of the flesh.

- In Summer: The Qi reaches the absolute surface, residing within the skin and the minute connecting vessels.

Autumn and Winter: Deep Needling During autumn and winter, Yang Qi moves downward and retreats deeper into the body's interior. To successfully reach the Qi and expel deeply lodged pathogens, needling must be deeper.

- In Autumn: The Qi begins to retreat and resides within the borders of the flesh.

- In Winter: The Qi sinks to its deepest levels, hiding within the sinews, bones, and marrow. Needles must be inserted deeply and retained for a longer period of time to access this deeply hidden Qi.

Three Talents

"First, the needle pierces to arrive inside the skin; thus it is called 'Heaven Talent'. Pause slightly and advance the needle, piercing within the human flesh; this is called 'Human Talent'. Once again pause and advance the needle, piercing to arrive between the sinew and bone; this is called 'Earth Talent'."
Ode to the Golden Needle, from Zhenjiu Dacheng

We can consider the three needling depths spoken of in the *Ling Shu*. What are these three depths?

The first depth is at the surface level of the skin layer. This is the Heavenly layer. This is the Yang level, like the sky or atmosphere of the body.

The second needling depth is located slightly deeper, in the flesh and muscle. This is the Human layer. This is the interface between the exterior and the interior.

The third needling depth is even deeper, at the level of the tendons and the bones. This is the Earthly layer. This is the internal, the innermost Yin of the body.

These three layers cover the entire spectrum of our being and of the cosmos. If we take them into account when applying our needling, we can reach the location of a disease at any level it resides. This is an application of the fractal-holographic cosmological view of the human body.

Needling Specific Tissues

Viewing the human body as a fractal system allows us to take advantage of inherent relationships in diagnosis and needling. The ancients understood intuitively that one could treat 'like with like' and so they organized phenomena in the world according to a theory of systematic correspondences.[1] The same resonances which they applied to the external world are reflected in human physiology.

According to the system of mutual correspondences, specific tissues have a resonant relationship to macrocosmic patterns of Qi embodied by Yin Yang and Wu Xing. As stated in the *Ling Shu*:

> *"The correlate of the heart are the vessels, its splendor appears in complexion, its rulers are the kidneys. The correlate of the lung is the skin, its splendor appears in the body hair, its ruler is the heart. The correlates of the liver are the sinews, its splendor appears in the nails, its ruler is the lung. The correlate of the spleen is the flesh, its splendor appears in the lips, its ruler is the liver. The correlates of the kidneys are the bones, their splendor is in the hair on the head, their ruler is the spleen."*
> *Su Wen, Chapter 10*

We can use these relationships to focus our acupuncture treatments, to choose our points more effectively, and to needle them more accurately for the best results. When possible, choosing points situated within specific tissues focuses the treatment effects according to our goals and strategy. This concept is related to and can be combined with the concept of needling depth.

For example, by needling into an area near a vessel or capillary bed, we are influencing the Fire and the Heart Qi of the patient. By needling shallowly at the skin surface, we are interacting with the Metal and the Lung Qi and the exterior. By needling into a tendon we are influencing the Wood and Liver Qi of the patient. By needling into the flesh and muscle we are influencing the Soil and the Spleen Qi. By needling deeply to tap a bone, we are engaging the Water and the Kidney Qi and the depths.

By engaging specific localized tissues with acupuncture, our actions influence and exert global effects due to the fractal nature of our physiology and the inherent resonant harmonies of Qi.

---

1. Medicine in China: A History of Ideas

Two Points, One Needle

If we can treat two points at once as a combination with one needle then all the better, as this would be a more powerful needle with a broader action and effect. By utilizing our intelligence when inserting a needle, we can visualize where it goes and point its internal trajectory towards a second point beyond the insertion site. By doing this, we can stimulate two points and thus two channels at the same time. Here are a few examples to get you started:

Needling *Zhong Bai* so that it stimulates the fascia underneath HT 8.

This stimulates both SJ and HT channels, which both synergize together as they both treat the GB and KD channels.

Needling SJ5 deeply so that it stimulates the fascia between PC6 or PC5.

This stimulates both the SJ and PC channels, creating a more potent treatment potential.

Needling LV3 towards KD1 so that it stimulates the fascia of the inner foot.

These are potential examples of ways to employ this concept. Using our creativity, many more can exist throughout the body. However, always be aware of contraindicated locations where deep needling can cause injury, or where an important vessel or structure is located. This method is really great to use on distal points on the limbs where there are clusters of points accessible with a single needle.

Venting & Transport Needling

"For shallow floating diseases, do not needle deeply."
Ling Shu, Chapter 3

The most superficial needling is at the very surface of the skin. It barely penetrates at all. Using a guide tube, just tap the needle in gently so that it stays but barely retains its sturdiness.

The surface of the skin is the most external part of our physiology. The ancients call the Qi which circulates here the Wei Qi. This is the most Yang protective and defensive Qi of our bodies. The skin and pores are the external entry points to our physiological system. They are the first line of defense to an often hostile external thermodynamic world which houses fierce molecular winds and external pathogens of various kinds. Our skin and Wei Qi are the frontier borderlands of our empire and immune system. From a fractal holographic perspective, shallow needling will treat the external layer. This is in line with the principles of superficial and deep needling.

The immune system and inflammation are intricately related and inseparable. They are also completely intertwined with the mental-emotional state of an organism. The spirit can be incensed or calm. The nervous system can be excited or relaxed. The immune system can be activated or at rest. If the spirit is incensed, if the nervous system is excited, or if the immune system is activated inappropriately, then we may consider using a venting technique.

Heat and inflammation are signs of a struggle between the body's defenses and a pathogenic influence. By venting, we can give this trapped heat and inflammation a pathway to escape and exit the surface level. Utilize the Back Shu points to vent from the Zang organs and their energetic ecosystems. The Shu points are frequently mentioned in the classics as areas of utmost importance for treatment. Erythema will form around the point as it vents inflammation.

Look at the patient's back. If there is visible red inflammation, such as redness or inflammation at the skin and surface, we may consider using the venting technique there. Observe the locations of points known for draining heat. Sometimes visible inflammation can be seen near points such as LI11, LU5, BL40, or GV15, for example.

Venting is by its nature a very gentle but dispersing technique which can help resolve issues which manifest as systemic inflammation, stress, and agitation. This by its nature is a form of drainage.

Electrical Needles

Humans are made of water and are electrically conductive beings. Muscles fire and move through electrical impulse and the exchange of ions. The nervous system and brain are a supercomputer of electrically charged chemical communication. Our physiology as a whole is a symphony of bio-electrochemical reactions working in sequence and harmony.

Having the ability to apply electrically modulating currents in targeted ways is a powerful acupuncture combination. The needle is able to penetrate and reach the inner depths of muscular, fascial or connective tissues. Sending electricity through the needle will cause a muscle to continually repolarize and twitch, essentially resetting it repeatedly. This can help chronically tense muscles to let go, or it can wake up muscles which have lost their ability to become consciously activated.

> *"Whether used alone to improve motor impairment or embedded within complex systems to create functional multi-joint movement, the potential that electrical stimulation holds for rehabilitation recovery is immeasura ble."*[1]

Different frequencies of electricity are also known to variably stimulate the nervous system. Neurochemicals are released for analgesic modulatory effect. Electricity applied to the needle can be a very effective tool for pain management. Acupuncture is a very precise treatment and the exact frequency and intensity of the electricity can be dialed in according to the therapeutic necessity.

Low frequency: (typically 2 Hz, sometimes up to ~10-15 Hz): Accelerates release of enkephalins, β-endorphin, and endomorphins. Analgesia is naloxone-reversible and mediated via μ/δ receptors.

High frequency: (typically 100 Hz): Selectively increases dynorphin A release, mediated via κ receptors. Often less naloxone-sensitive at spinal levels for certain effects.

Intermediate frequencies: (e.g., 40-60 Hz): Can promote simultaneous or enhanced release of enkephalin, β-endorphin, and dynorphin in various CNS regions, sometimes yielding stronger analgesia in certain models.

Combined/alternating: (e.g., 2/100 Hz dense-disperse wave): Releases all four major EOPs (enkephalin, β-endorphin, endomorphin, dynorphin) with synergistic analgesic effects.[2]

I tend to use electrical stimulation acupuncture as a fallback method for difficult and stubborn cases of pain, or for muscle weakness and flaccidity.

---

1. Neuromuscular Electrical Stimulation for Skeletal Muscle Function
2. Acupuncture and endorphins

Obtaining the Qi

Dé Qì 得氣

"The acupuncturist must obtain the Qi (De Qi). If Qi has arrived, fastidiously hold it and do not lose it."
Ling Shu, Chapter 3

A concept that breathes life into one's acupuncture treatments, De Qi translates as 'obtaining' Qi. It is also sometimes referred to as the 'arrival' of the Qi. It is the sensation associated with a successful acupuncture treatment because it signals recognition by the body of the activation of the Qi and the physiological system of the patient. It can be a subjective sensation felt by the patient, and/or an objective reflexive reaction by the patient's body which is observed by the practitioner.

"Their Qì's arrival is like the appearance of a pulsing vessel. Follow the needle and pierce it. Obtain the Qì to push it inwards. This is called supplementation. To move and open it up, this is called drainage."
Nan Jing, Chapter 78

The patient may experience it in forms such as a twinging reaction, a heavy dullness or ache, a nerve-like sensation, electricity, tingling or numbness, feelings of movement or flowing of energy, warmth, cold, etc. The sensation will differ depending upon the nature of the point. Sensations vary with each point's nature such as its depth, its types of local tissues, or its energetic role. Learn these nuances to master their subtlety and sharpen one's treatments.

"The arrival of the Qi resembles the flocking together of crows."
Zhang Jeibin

The goal is not to elicit the strongest sensation possible. The goal is to activate the Qi of a living being on a whole-system level by stimulating a relevant point of physiological importance.

"Only when the Qi is reached, will acupuncture be effective. This effect, it is said, is as if the winds blow away the clouds and clear the azure sky."
Ling Shu, Chapter 1

Take care in handling the Qi of a human being, your patient. Overstimulation can be counterproductive. Be soft, yet firm; relaxed, yet focused. Tune your touch, as some patients need gentleness, while others thrive on a bolder surge of Qi.

The sensation of the arrival of the Qi should not be confused with the type of sharp pain which occurs at the superficial skin surface level. "Obtaining Qi is a deeper sensation, duller in nature, and less localized than the sharp pain associated with the stimulation of subcutaneous nerves."[1]

Sometimes it can be a challenge to obtain the Qi. On the Spleen channel, where dampness, as a heavy, stagnant energy, can bog down the Qi, obtaining it may prove elusive. At times, it may feel like an 'vacant house' when the patient is deficient here. Use rotation or thrusting to find it and stir it awake.

---

1. A Practical Dictionary of Chinese Medicine

Supplementation and Drainage

> *"All use of acupuncture is thus: to tonify hollowness, to disperse fullness, to dredge stasis; the evil to be overcome will thus weaken."*
> *Ling Shu, Chapter 1*

Supplementation and drainage methods are core to classical acupuncture practice. The Classics describe a number of different ways to carry this out. For one such method of supplementation and drainage, we use needle techniques involving varying speeds of insertion or withdrawal of the needle. One aspect of this method is outlined in the *Ling Shu*:

> *"Generally speaking, needling methods, 'slow then quick' produces tonification, 'quick then slow' produces dispersion."*
> *Ling Shu, Chapter 1*

A point which needs to be supplemented due to deficiency should be entered with slow deliberateness while simultaneously rotating the needle inwards. Envision the Qi travelling through the channel and entering the point; continue until the proper depth is reached and the Qi arrives at the point. If the Qi is not reached, then quickly exit the needle, but not all the way, just to the entrance, and enter slowly again while rotating. Repeat this process until the Qi arrives. This is related to needle grasp and De Qi. One of the goals of supplementation is to activate and gather the healthy Zheng Qi of the patient.

Sometimes we have to 'fish' for the Qi if it is very weakened, repressed, depleted or hidden. This can happen when there is severe vacuity, dampness and phlegm or excess adipose tissue. Needling into emptiness is said to feel like a vacant hall. Some exemplary points for this type of supplementation technique are SP6, SP8, SP9, ST 36, LI10, LV3, or CV6, CV10.

A point which needs to be drained due to excess should be entered quickly into the body to the desired depth of the tissue, if the point allows for it. Once inserted, remove the point with slow deliberateness while simultaneously rotating the needle outwards. Envision Qi leaving the point and the channel with the needle. These two techniques are essentially opposite mirrors of each other. Some exemplary points for this type of drainage technique are LI11, LV3, LU5, ST40, SJ5 or GB30.

> *"The unskilled physician grasps only the form when they use the techniques of acupuncture. The superior physician understands the spirit of humanity includes both the Blood and Qi, whether there is an excess or deficiency, whether he should tonify or disperse."*
> *Ling Shu, Chapter 3*

These techniques can be applied to any needled point, including Dao Mao groups, and be interchanged depending upon the context. A primary goal is for the Qi to arrive. Then we can make the decision to either supplement it and guide it deeper or to drain it and release it; to concentrate it or guide it out.

> *"Supplementation and draining must not be carried out at random; they should match heaven and earth as if it were one with them. Grasp the nature of this oneness to know death and survival."*
> *Su Wen, Chapter 17*

We need to be clear in our diagnosis and our treatment strategy so that we can execute a focused and rational plan. A point which is supplemented in one patient may then be required to be drained on the next patient. Many points are flexible in that way. Other points work best as a supplementation point or a drainage point. By learning the nature of each point, we can learn when to utilize them and why, and with the best techniques. It is not uncommon to use *both* supplementation and drainage in one treatment. Outside of excessive heat disorders, this is explicitly recommended by some:

> *"...only balanced supplementation and drainage is suitable. One must first drain, then supplement. This is called 'first draining evil Qì, then supplementing true Qì'. This is the secret formula not passed on by the earlier masters."*
> *Supplementation and Drainage of the Classic of Spiritual Correspondence, from the Zhenjiu Dacheng*

The way in which we remove the needle is another important factor which influences whether an action supplements or drains. This is stressed repeatedly in the classics. For example, after supplementation one should close the needle hole and stop the true Qi from leaking out.

> *"When needling is complete, use the hand to stroke and close their acupoint, like righteously applying earth to fill it up... After withdrawing the needle, use the hand to stroke and close their acupoint, causing the Qì to not leak out."*
> *Ode of Mysterious Indications, from the Zhenjiu Dacheng*

In contrast, after drainage, one might allow the point to remain unclosed, to give the pathogen or evil a route to escape through and leave.

> *"With exhalation, slowly, slowly withdraw the needle. Do not close their acupoint, this is called 'drainage'."*
> *Supplementation and Drainage of Master Gāo of Sìmíng, from the Zhenjiu Dacheng*

These quotes illustrate that the art of needling does not cease when the needle enters the body, or even after manipulation or De Qi, but continues even through the act of needle removal and how we interact with the acupuncture point after removal.

Open or Closed

"The spirit, ah! The spirit guest is located at the gates."
The Ode of Mysterious Indications, from the Zhenjiu Dacheng

After we needle, acupuncture points can remain open or they can be closed. We must remember, these are gates, portals, holes, through which Qi can either escape or enter. We must be able to guard the portals, guard the gates for a patient who is deficient, to prevent pathogens from entering. We must also allow pathogens a route to exit for patients who are excess. Guarding the gates guards the spirit of the patient.

"'The spirit guest' means the upright and the evil share a common meeting place. 'The spirit' means the upright Qì. 'The guest' means the evil Qì. 'At the gates' means the evil Qì follows the places where the upright Qì exists and enters."
Supplementation and Drainage of the Inner Classic, from the Zhenjiu Dacheng

What is allowed to pass through the gates contributes to the methods of supplementation and drainage. Do not let a weakened, deficient patient's blood and Qi escape, and do not let external wind or evils enter through the acupuncture holes which you used to treat them. This is done by closing their acupuncture point. I do this by firmly pressing or stroking the point with a cotton ball. But for a patient with an excess disorder who is being drained, one can allow the pathogen to leave through the hole first as a little bit of blood, and then close it to guard their upright Qi. For this reason, treatment doesn't just stop when the needles go in. The treatment continues and clinical decisions are to be made even after the needles are removed!

Blood Letting

If Blood becomes stagnant, pain and symptoms of disease will result. Stagnation creates inflammation and sludgy flows, impeding the natural flow of the fractal physiological river basin of blood and creating blockages in tissues. Of course, if this occurs inside of a major artery or blood vessel it is life-threatening. But it can also happen within the micro-cellular environments throughout the entire ecosystem of the body, such as in the fascia. This results in pain, structural damage, and debilitated function.

> *"When the blood is replete [stagnant], one must open it [blood-let]."*
> *Su Wen, Chapter 5*

Cupping (and gua sha) are potent methods for directly treating stagnant blood (and sha). But acupuncture can also release blood stagnation via blood letting. Blood letting is explicitly a drainage method for clearing excesses, such as heat or blood stagnation. Since ancient times, the act of blood letting has been recommended as a potent treatment for helping to resolve issues involving stagnant blood. The way to find areas of blood letting is to use our observational, diagnostic, and clinical skills. Look for dark capillaries or ashen webs — these serve as visual marks indicating blood stagnation — and prick these branches to release the stagnant blood in the Jingluo. Points such as BL40, PC3, GV14, BL17, KD2, or the ear apex are some examples of places to consider blood letting.[1]

> *"Observe where the blood is and take it."*
> *Wang Bing*

It is critical for the acupuncturist to remove blockages and blood stagnation from tissues. Doing so will restore proper flow and enable the body's healing capacities. Just like flowing water will restore a barren ecosystem, allowing the return of fresh blood to stagnant areas will restore the local physiological environments. Change and transformation will be reflected by subtle changes in color to the area and the collaterals.

> *"One must first remove an evil from the blood vessels, and only then one regulates any depletion or repletion. Regardless which disease is concerned, the treatment is continued until a balance is reached."*
> *Su Wen, Chapter 20*

Bloodletting[2] removes blockages and releases the excess detritus causing the stagnation. It opens up a pathway for the life-giving fluids and blood of the body to reenter those previously blocked-off physiological spaces for microenvironment regeneration. Removing small amounts of stagnancy, despite being a form of drainage, can in fact be supplementing by enabling better Qi and blood flow, and by stimulating metabolic and cellular function.

Pathogens and waste can be cleared from the body by evicting the stagnant blood. This includes heat and inflammation, which can be very useful for many different scenarios. For this reason, the well and the spring points are sometimes chosen, particularly in the Spring and Summer.

---

1. Bleeding Peripheral Points: An Acupuncture Technique

2. Pricking the Vessels: Bloodletting Therapy in Chinese Medicine

External Essays

The essays in this section pertain to topics related to knowledge, theory, practice, concepts, and ideas. I think of these as the Yang essays of the book. Traditional concepts and theories which are foundational to the practice of acupuncture are written about. My own concepts, theories and ideas are also formulated.

Qi Holes

Xué 穴

"Those which are called acupuncture points refer to the place where the spirit Qi and its flowing movement, in and out, is unhampered by skin, flesh, muscle, or bone."
Ling Shu, Chapter 1

Acupuncture points are represented by the Chinese character *xué*. Etymologically, this character "reflects the notion that acupuncture points are usually depressions or crevices between bones, sinews, etc."[1] They can be thought of like 'Qi holes'; areas where the Qi, flowing like rivers through a water basin, forms natural eddies in the ceaseless current. It conforms to the logic of the landscape; the anatomy of the human organism.

Human bodies all fundamentally share the same principle. So these holes are the physiologically active zones of the human body. Oftentimes, they are areas dense and rich in surrounding connective, circulatory, or neurological structures. These zones pulse with life—nerve endings, blood vessels, and fascia intertwine here, letting us engage the full spectrum of Qi and ripple its effects cascading throughout the body.

"The interstices of the flesh are locations of interaction. These locations of interaction have the names of needling holes."
Zhang Zhicong

---

1. A Practical Dictionary of Chinese Medicine

Qi Sensations

When Qi is attained, each point invokes its own particular sensation. The classics describe De Qi as aching, dull, heavy, numbness, warmth, or coldness. Of De Qi it is said that "it is a special sensation between pleasant and outright pain, or tolerable dull pain for patients, therefore, sharp pain should not be included."[1]

Research suggests that the various De Qi sensations can relate to the activation of different afferent nerve fibers.[2] This reflects the structure and functions of each particular point. The entire connective tissue matrix of our body is innervated and communicating with our nervous system. Qi holes are specifically located in areas of high physiological reactivity. Acupuncture therefore triggers a physiological phenomenon in the peripheral and central nervous system and De Qi is an indication of this cascading whole-body physiological event.

Not every sensation is associated with De Qi, however. Sharp pain, which occurs at the skin surface, is specifically to be avoided. Research has shown the effects which De Qi has on various brain structures as well as neuromatrixes related to pain. This effect, however, is negated and perhaps even reversed if one causes sharp pain at the skin surface.[3]

The successful acupuncturist must practice and master the skill of attaining the Qi at the various depths, but without aggravating the pain receptors at the surface. With purpose, clarity, and focus, strike true to find the Qi and elicit the proper sensation.

> *"In acupuncture, one must hit the Qi holes and not attack the flesh or its sections. In hitting the Qi hole, the needling causes the Qi to flow in the passages. Attacking the flesh and the sections will pain the skin."*
> *Ling Shu, Chapter 4*

---

1. Acupuncture De Qi: From Characterization to Underlying Mechanism

2. Ibid.

3. A Literature Review of De Qi in Clinical Studies

Needle Grasp

'Needle grasp' is an important aspect of the De Qi phenomenon. This refers to the grasping effect which takes place by the body onto the needle when the Qi has been attained. The classics portray this vividly:

> *"The acupuncturist may feel as though the needle is being firmly grabbed and moving roughly when the Qi arrives, but only loosely grasped and moving smoothly if the Qi does not arrive. Qi arrival feels like a fish biting a hook and bobbing in the water; if Qi does not arrive, the acupuncturist feels as though the needle is in a quiet empty house."*
> *Ode to Mysterious Indications, from the Zhenjiu Dacheng*

Needle grasp is related to the interaction between the needle and the various connective tissues and fascia. When a needle is inserted, and especially when it is rotated or manipulated in various ways, the connective tissue fibers wind around the needle. This grasping of the needle "transmits a mechanical signal to connective tissue cells via mechanotransduction."[1] It can be instantaneous, seen as an involuntary fasciculation. Sometimes, it requires stimulation in order for the body's Qi to grasp the needle.

These mechanical signals ripple through the entire organism, carried by the ubiquitous, system-wide communication network of the fascia and connective tissue. Needle manipulation and needle techniques such as rotation, thrusting, or lifting, help to coax the fascia into engaging. I think of the fascia as a meta-communication network which is tapped in directly to the central controls of our physiology. When the body grasps the needle, the De Qi sensation and needle grasp phenomenon is a way of saying *'signal received!'*

De Qi is the basis for the physiological modulatory cascade which occurs as a result of acupuncture. In my experience, attaining contact with the Qi is the essential component of acupuncture — without it, the healing effect is not as potently engaged. When the Qi has been attained, the signal has been both sent and received. Physiological contact has been made: the 'fish bites the hook' and a profound modulatory cascade is underway.

---

1. Mechanical signaling through connective tissue: a mechanism for the therapeutic effect of acupuncture

Acupuncture Dosage

Does acupuncture have a dosage? And if so, can this be measured?

Acupuncture can be strong or it can be light. It can be powerful, as well as gentle. Different needling techniques will have different effects. Some reach into the depths and surge Qi powerfully, while others softly vent the surface and exterior. The way we engage with the Qi through our needle techniques, coupled with the focus and intention of our Spirit, ultimately determines the relative strength of the acupuncture 'dose'.

One way in which 'dosage' has been observed and measured is by scientifically monitoring the brain function and nervous system fluctuations in a patient receiving acupuncture. Measuring the fMRI alterations in neural networks yields information about how neurophysiologically intense the Qi reacts to the treatment. The Triple-needle 'Dao Ma' acupuncture technique achieves a stronger effect compared to a single needle, or a single needle with twirling and thrusting techniques applied to it.[1] Such research underscores the Triple-needle 'Dao Ma' technique's potency and is part of why I consider it to be a foundational needling strategy.

In normal clinical situations we do not have the ability to observe neuromatrix brain responses. We rely on subtler tools: a clear, attentive mind and a honed Spirit which is attuned to the patient's Qi through subtle observation. If the Spirit is honed, clear, and quiescent, we will be able to notice even the slightest De Qi reaction, let alone a strong response. If there is no response, then we know that the Qi has not been reached and a meaningful dose has not yet been applied.

Sometimes, a stronger dose is appropriate. Other times, a gentle touch can be more effective. Understanding the context of the situation requires careful observation so that we can be in tune with the Qi of the patient and the practical goals of the treatment. If someone is sensitive, be gentle. If someone is strong, be firm. However, it is essential for the Qi to arrive in a meaningful dose for the healing response to be engaged.

1. Effect of acupuncture 'dose' on modulation of the default mode network of the brain.

A Pole Casting a Shadow

"On understanding the moving power and its Way: the onset of a therapeutic effect is like an arrow striking its target, and nothing can withstand it."
Ling Shu, Chapters 1 and 38[1]

A pole hit by the sun immediately casts its shadow.[2] Similarly, acupuncture should immediately cast its effects. If there is no observable effect and neither the patient nor the acupuncturist can detect a response, then can we really say that we have done anything? If the Qi does not arrive, how can anything be expected to happen?

When we yell into a canyon, we should be greeted by an echo. This is how we know when we have reached the Qi, as it will greet us with a response.

"The Way of Nature is like an echo responding to a sound."
Wen Zi, Chapter 69

We must grasp the Qi in order to have an effect. When it arrives, the body will echo its response and let us know when this has been achieved in various ways. Either the patient will feel it or the practitioner will sense it. Subtle movements, the firing of muscle, the formation of redness; if we are subtle we will observe the body's echo. With De Qi there will be an effect, just as a pole placed in the sun inevitably casts its shadow.

"When the Qi is reached, there will be an effect."
Ling Shu, Chapter 9

The Ling Shu describes acupuncture as a trigger, but the inner mechanism is the Qi. By understanding the Qi we will know how to activate the trigger properly. If we don't understand the Qi, then we are blindly fumbling about for the trigger to an obscure and potentially misunderstood mechanism. As with a firearm or a crossbow, it is irresponsible to recklessly fire this trigger. Know the entire mechanism so that we can activate the trigger effectively and responsibly.

> *"The unrefined practitioners guard the trigger. Outstanding practitioners guard the inner mechanism."*
> *Ling Shu, Chapter 1*

---

1. This quote is a paraphrase which combines elements of both chapters.
2. This image comes from an ancient technique of setting up a vertical pole in sunlight to observe its shadow length and direction. This was used for timekeeping, determining solstices/equinoxes, and forming the calendar.

Effects Over Time

Generally acupuncture should have an immediate effect, like a pole casting a shadow, or a noise returning an echo. But it also has effects which occur over time. It initiates a systemic, cascading process which then unfolds multidimensionally throughout the entire fractal physiological network of the patient.

The internal environments of the body exist on many different time and size scales, from the microcosmic levels of molecular and cellular landscapes, up through to the organs all the way to the macrocosmic realities of our physical body and mental emotional experience.

Events take time to play out and transpire amidst the multiple levels of this overwhelming physiological complexity, and thus acupuncture's effects ripple out in time after a treatment. It is like throwing a rock into a lake. There is an initial splash, but then there are concentric ripples which reverberate for a period of time afterwards as the multitudinous, distributed effects and feedback loops all respond to the stimulation and issue forth throughout the unified organismic whole.

After the treatment has been completed and positive effects have occurred, how long will they last? Part of this depends on whether the root of the issue was resolved. Some diseases have deeper roots than others. Lifestyle, habits, and the daily practices of a patient can either work against or contribute to the positive inertia of an acupuncture treatment. Research suggests that a successful treatment of chronic pain with acupuncture can persist for a long time, with a time horizon of at least a year.[1]

---

1. The persistence of the effects of acupuncture after a course of treatment: A meta-analysis of patients with chronic pain.

Point Combinations

With herbs, it is common practice to combine a pair of medicines in order to create a powerful synergy which is more effective than the sum of its parts. This is called 'Dui Yao' in the tradition of Chinese herbal medicine. This way of thinking can also be applied to acupuncture point selection. We can think of points in this way, and should strive to continually develop new combinations. Powerful combinations of points are like effective keys to complex locks.

Commonly, powerful combinations can be developed by simply thinking logically about what we are treating. Where is the pain? What is the sick channel? By applying correct diagnosis, we then create an opportunity for the creative development of a powerful and effective point combination. This is the treatment. Utilizing distal points on the opposite side or end of the body, on channels which we know through Jing Luo channel theory to have a connection to the sick channel, we can discover powerful and unique ways to apply acupuncture effectively to any unique situation.

Channel theory offers a natural method for devising synergistic point combinations by utilizing various natural interconnections between the channels. These relationships are understood in terms of the mathematics of Chinese natural philosophies such as Yin Yang, Wu Xing, and the Ba Gua. This is the rationale behind many treatment methods and styles of acupuncture, such as the systems used by Dr. Tan.

Less is More

"Those who know beginning and end, they make one statement, and that is enough."
Ling Shu, Chapter 5

If we have a clear diagnosis of the situation, then we can deduce a straightforward strategy. A convoluted or overly complex treatment is an indication that there may be confusion in either one's diagnosis or treatment strategy. A focused treatment plan and articulatable needle selection indicates that there is clear reason and intention behind what is being done. More needles does not necessarily equate to more results. We cannot brute force healing to occur. Focus instead on making each needle count the most. Attain the Qi and use good technique.

"The Master does his job and then stops. He understands that the universe is forever out of control, and that trying to dominate events goes against the current of the Dao."
Dao De Jing, Chapter 30

Just as in speech where 'those who know say little and those who are ignorant never stop speaking'[1], an acupuncture treatment that is concise is potent and quietly 'says volumes without speaking'. If we needle every point and send 1000 different signals to the body simultaneously, how can it be expected to be able to receive the correct transmission amidst all the noise? If everyone is talking all at once and yelling over each other, is it possible for proper communication to take place? A treatment like this can be likened to playing a piano by hitting every piano key simultaneously.

"In the pursuit of knowledge, everyday something is added. In the pursuit of the Dao, everyday something is dropped."
Dao De Jing, Chapter 48

Strive to be intentional. Make each needle count. Acupuncture can be as simple as Yin and Yang — there is no need to overcomplicate things. Trust in the value of the work, in the nature of the medicine to achieve its goals, and in the wisdom of the body to respond appropriately. Bringing this mindset, construct each treatment with purpose. Strive towards what is necessary and remove excess or filler. Then step back and allow it to work.

"If you want to accord with the Dao, just do your job, then let go."
Dao De Jing, Chapter 24

A great way to develop intentional point selection is to limit the amount of points we allow ourselves to use during a single treatment. The practice of distilling one's treatment strategy down to the most essential points for the given clinical context will train the acupuncturist to make the most out of each point and each decision. First try only using the ten needles from one single needle package. Then, see if you can distill your treatment strategy to only four points, or even two points. We can ask ourselves, if we had only one single point available to treat this patient beautifully, what would it be? Even if we only do this as a thought experiment, the practice of doing so is profound and beneficial to our practice.[2]

---

1. Dao De Jing, Chapter 56

2. See the book *One Needle Therapy: Pain Syndromes.*

Wind

Fēng 風

The fact is, the wind is the origin of a hundred illnesses. In case a person is clear and calm, the flesh and the interstice structures are firmly closed up and resist."
Su Wen, Chapter 3

Wind is often considered a conceptual precursor in the development of the concept of Qi.[1] We can think of wind as the spontaneous physical manifestation of Qi in motion. It is one of the most primordial forces of the human experience. All of our ancestors experienced the wind, whether as a gentle breeze or as a terrifying and destructive storm.

Wind results from the interaction between cold and heat in the environment causing pressure differentials. Temperature gradients emerge because the Sun does not heat the surfaces of the Earth uniformly due to differences in how the varying complex surfaces (ex: mountains, lakes, plains) absorb and radiate heat. Warmer air expands, becoming less dense, and thus rises, creating areas of lower pressure near the ground where it was. Conversely, cooler air contracts, becoming denser, and sinks, forming high-pressure areas. The air in high pressure areas rapidly flows to the areas of low pressure and this movement is what we experience as wind. Wind therefore represents a fundamental expression of Yin and Yang and the thermodynamic flow of Qi in nature.

Living organisms constantly produce energy through metabolic processes like cellular respiration. This energy production maintains our internal conditions (like temperature, pH, and ion concentrations) so that they are different from the external environment. It is essential to life that we keep our internal thermodynamics from reaching complete equilibrium with the environment, which is the thermodynamic equivalent to death. For this purpose, life developed semi-permeable membranes such as the skin and cellular membranes. These barriers manage the flows of energy and matter between the internal and external environments, preventing thermodynamic dissipation of the organism.

> *"When the nutritive and defensive [Qì] diffuse and flow then one attains favorable results."*
> *Ode of the Twelve-Step Manual Method, from the Zhenjiu Dacheng*

In terms of Chinese medicine, this barrier membrane function relates to the Wei Qi, also known as the Defensive or Guard Qi, which metaphorically guards the barriers and borderlands of the empire to make sure that invaders do not enter and pillage the vulnerable interior Ying Qi, the Valley or Constructive Qi. This is the Yin and Yang of the exterior and the interior of the organism. The Yang exterior of the organism is fundamentally engaged in a continual thermodynamic regulatory struggle with the Wind. Whereas the more vulnerable Yin interior is engaged with the necessary metabolic and generative functions that maintain life and its growth and nourishment at the various different organ and cellular levels.

> *"Wind is the chief of the one hundred diseases. When it comes to changes and transformations, other diseases result. It has no permanent cardinal point where it comes from. However, whatever sets in does so because of Wind Qi."*
> *Su Wen, Chapter 42*

It is essential for the body to maintain its thermodynamic integrity in the face of hostile thermodynamic forces such as wind. Necessary inner life processes of the organism must proceed uninterrupted and without disruption. It is believed that if wind can penetrate the exterior portions of the body, it will often carry other pathogenic factors. When Wind pierces the exterior, it also sweeps in cold or damp, igniting an inflammatory struggle. Ultimately, the ensuing physiological dysregulation this causes results in a multitude of illnesses. For this reason, wind is considered the 'origin or chief of the hundred illnesses'.

The body has mechanisms such as sweating, vasodilation, or shivering in order to spontaneously regulate the exterior. This regulation prevents rapid loss of thermal energy to the environment and is useful to expel pathogens. Therefore, treatment strategies for

Wind often involve acupuncture points or herbal formulas which regulate and influence these exterior portions of the body.

Consider the pathological patterns and formulas described in such detail in the *Shang Han Lun*.[2] Formulas such as *Ma Huang Tang* and *Gui Zhi Tang* are representative of the strategy of activating the exterior to purge wind-related illnesses. By assisting the body in expelling pathogens from the exterior, homeostasis can be restored. We might consider as a thought experiment which points would correlate to these herbal strategies from a purely acupuncture perspective. I think that reverse-engineering herbal formulas into acupuncture protocols is a great learning practice.

Points Correlating to the Strategy of Ma Huang Tang (Exterior Repletion/Wind-Cold):

Ma Huang Tang is the representative formula for cold damage (exterior repletion), characterized by wind-cold fettering the exterior, severe generalized pain, inhibited lung Qi (panting), and an absence of sweating.

- LI4: This is a primary point used to expel wind-cold and release the exterior. Crucially, it is classically indicated for chills and fever that are accompanied by an absence of sweating, which perfectly aligns with the *Ma Huang Tang* presentation of wind-cold.

- LU7: Often combined with LI4 when exterior wind invades the body, LU7 assists in expelling the pathogen while restoring the descending and disseminating functions of the Lungs. This directly mirrors *Ma Huang Tang*'s secondary function to "diffuse the lung and calm panting" when the exterior is blocked.

- BL11: Located on the upper back, this point has a strong action on the exterior portion of the body and is used to expel wind-cold that manifests as stiffness and pain of the neck, cold shivering, and the absence of sweating.

Points Correlating to the Strategy of *Gui Zhi Tang* (Exterior Vacuity/Wind Strike):

Gui Zhi Tang is the primary formula for wind strike (exterior vacuity), characterized by an insecure defensive exterior where the construction-yin (nutritive qi) is not contained, leading to spontaneous sweating and a disharmony between construction and defense.

- BL12 (Wind Gate): This point directly mirrors the *Gui Zhi Tang* strategy. It is explicitly indicated for patterns of exterior deficiency where a wind attack causes a "disharmony of nutritive Qi and defensive Qi," presenting with fever, chills, an aversion to wind, and sweating that fails to relieve the condition.

- DU16 (Palace of Wind) & GB20 (Wind Pool): These points are explicitly linked to *Gui Zhi Tang* in Zhang Zhong-jing's *Shang Han Lun*. The classical text instructs that if a patient with a Taiyang disorder is given *Gui Zhi Tang* and experiences agitation, the practitioner should first needle GB20 and DU16, and then re-prescribe *Gui Zhi Tang* to achieve a cure. Furthermore, DU16 is specifically applied to treat the exact Taiyang wind pattern of disharmony of the nutritive Qi and defensive Qi accompanied by sweating.

---

1. A Vision of the Origin of Qi Through Wind and Flavours

2. Shang Han Lun, The Treatise on Cold Damage

Qì

Qì 氣

"That which genuinely exists in the universe is only the existential process from what has shape to the shapeless, and from the shapeless to what has shape. And this is just the dynamism of Qi. This conception of the dynamism of Qi synthesizes the concepts of being and nothingness, and the concrete and empty."
Zhang Zai

At its most foundational level, Qi is the primordial, psycho-physical stuff of the universe, simultaneously encompassing both matter and energy, structure and function. The universe is an organismic process driven by the perpetual transformations of Qi. All entities come into physical existence through the condensation of Qi and, upon death or destruction, disintegrate as their Qi disperses back into the formless void.

Everything in our lives exists in relation to the sun's Qi. The days are a result of the earth's rotation, as its seasons are of its revolution around the sun. We experience these as temporal sine waves of Qi, and everything which is occurring on the planet is a result of fluctuating availability of the sun's Qi.

The character for Qi graphically depicts vapors originating from rice. Etymologically, its original and most common meaning refers to gaseous substances like vapor, steam, breath, or air. We can relate to the concrete image of steam rising from fresh-cooked rice being generalized and abstracted by philosophers and medical practitioners into the fundamental, life-sustaining material force that animates the universe.

Qi functions as an existential concept because it represents the fundamental ground of actualization, the synthesis of being and non-being, and the dynamic continuity of life and death. From an existential standpoint, if Qi does not exist, then there cannot be any actual thing at all. The universe then can be understood as an existential process moving perpetually between being and non-being, existence and non-existence, Qi and no Qi.

In this sense, Qi transforms the existential understanding of death from a terrifying abyss of absolute annihilation into a natural phase of cosmic continuity. Qi frames existence not as a static state of "being," but as an active, continuous project of "becoming." The cosmos, understood through Qi, is a spontaneously self-generating organismic process characterized by continuity, wholeness, and dynamism. Human existence is inextricably embedded in this organic web, and we ourselves are active participants in the ongoing process.

True and Proper

Zhèng 正

The Chinese character *Zhèng* can be translated as what is true, proper, upright, or principled. As a verb, it is to correct something, or to rectify it. To be Zhèng is to act appropriately and timely. In philosophy, Zhèng can be applied to the moral actions of the individual. In this sense it is something righteous or upright. In medicine, Zhèng can also be applied to the functions of the body and to the Qi.

Physiologically, when something is working properly, efficiently, and effectively, this is Zhèng Qi. The normally functioning Qi of the body, when harmonious and proper, can be said to be healthy. Zhèng Qi is therefore the Qi of the system functioning properly and appropriately for the benefit of the organism's life. It is a system which is able to maintain its stability and closure in the face of the endless threat of thermodynamic dissipation, invasion by external pathogens, or internal chaos and collapse.

Qi which acts in opposition to Zhèng Qi was referred to as evil Qi by the ancient Chinese. This is Qi which is not acting harmoniously, not behaving properly, and is disrupting the efficient operations of a healthy physiological system. It could be chaotic Qi from the external environment, or it could be due to malfunctioning processes internally. "Right Qi stands in opposition to evil Qi, which is any entity in its active aspect of harming the body."[1]

We could imagine an example of this in the case of an autoimmune inflammatory disease, where the body's own immune system, acting perversely, attacks itself. This is improper functioning, akin to a rebellion. An empire in rebellion is neither healthy nor strong, but rather teeters into chaos. Authority of the emperor wanes, civil strife and banditry occurs, and the continuity of the state and the society is in jeopardy. Therefore, the purpose of acupuncture is to correct and rectify the Qi, to make it Zhèng, and to support it to remain proper and organized in the face of hostile forces both within and without. Physiological unity must remain intact, organized, and upright for health to flourish.

"If one governs his person by complying with the ordering principle of things, life will be kept intact."
The Annals of Lü Buwei, Book 5 Chapter 4.1

---

1. A Practical Dictionary of Chinese Medicine

Visitors and Guests

Kè 客

Life by definition stands in thermodynamic opposition to the external environment. Through energetic exchange, life continually strives to increase and maintain the internal order of its systems despite the tendency for energy to dissipate and disorder to increase over time. In this way, living beings are engaged in a continual struggle and interface with their environment and ultimately, with the energetic and thermodynamic realities of the universe.

The second law of thermodynamics states that entropy will always increase in any system over time. Life then has developed the unique ability to maintain an out-of-equilibrium stability, a unity and dynamic order, in the face of this second law.

External barriers and semi-permeable interfaces such as the skin, cellular membranes, and the boundary closures of living structures, enable the delicate thermodynamic dance of life to continue through continual energy exchange. "Biological systems are thermodynamic open (dissipative) systems, traversed by a continuous flow of matter and energy; yet on the other hand, they realize closure."[1] This energy exchange is essential to the maintenance of life, but it also comes with potential dangers.

The Zheng Qi is the energy of the living system which works to maintain order and stability. It is the Qi of the living host, analogous to the Qi of a state. Any Qi which runs counter to this purpose, whether internally or externally, can be considered an unwelcome visitor or guest in the system, a form of evil Qi.

Much like a state receives guests, emissaries, diplomats, and foreign dignitaries, a human body is also in contact with outsiders. Modern science is quite familiar with various types of pathogens which cause chaos, disorder, and increase the dissipative tendency of the living system. These are potentially agents of chaos which can cause rebellion or push the system towards disintegration.

> *"As for [guests/visitors], [the wind and the cold] arrive from outside like visitors; where they settle is not their permanent [residence]."*
> *Jang Jeibin*

When the Zheng Qi is strong, the living system and its functions are ordered, efficient, and effective. The borders of the organism and the empire are guarded and firm; it is more difficult for invaders to enter and create disruption. The Wei Qi, which is the defensive Qi of the body, functions properly. This is like a properly functioning immune system of the body, or the alert, loyal frontier guards of an empire. But if the Zheng Qi is depleted and weak, then the borders of the organism are open vulnerable and there will be more opportunities for incursions by hostile pathogens and environmental forces, like wind, cold, or microorganisms.

> *"When the body is exerted and sweat flows and when the interstice structures are open and meet with depletion wind, then the [latter] 'strikes man in a very subtle manner."*
> *Su Wen, Chapter 26*

For this reason, it is important to 'guard the gates'. It is necessary to keep the Zheng Qi of the body strong so that there are no areas of vulnerability to external attack. Wind strikes where the body is vulnerable in a very subtle manner. It is like an ambush by an enemy force. If attacked, the normal flow of Qi becomes disrupted and order turns to disorder. If allowed to continue, the problem can spread and amplify, becoming a hostile force setting up camp and attacking and raiding from within your own territory. Acupuncture can be used to remedy this situation by removing the hostile entity and reestablishing harmony.

> *"All these locations where the guard Qi can come to a halt and where the evil Qi can settle as a visitor. Needles and pointed stones remove the evil Qi in an encircling manner."*
> *Su Wen, Chapter 10*

The best way to treat illness is to prevent it from occurring. If illness does occur, it must be identified quickly. Hence, the *Su Wen* states that "the superior practitioner stops its sprouts, the inferior practitioner stops what has already fully developed." But if an unsavory guest does arrive, acupuncture can be extremely effective in expelling it. If it is new to the body, it floats aimlessly among the superficial Yang layers without a fixed location. Vent it, drain it, and guide it out before it sets up camp to become deeply anchored and chronic within.

> *"When the evil has come as a new visitor, it has no definite location yet. If one pushes it, it will move forward; if one pulls it, then it will stop. If one drains it as soon as one encounters it, this disease will come to an end at once."*
> *Su Wen, Chapter 27*

---

1. Biological Organisation as a Closure of Constraints.

Evil

Xié 邪

"Evil is a term for what is not proper."
Yang's Commentary, Nan Jing

Life in general is a tenuous proposition in a universe which tends towards thermodynamic equilibrium. Living beings, however, live outside of thermodynamic equilibrium in a semi-contained state of dynamic non-equilibrium. They house an ongoing, orderly, complex chemical process within their boundaries. The ability to maintain internal order and keep this thermodynamic and electro-chemical process going is the difference between life and its opposite, the static equilibrium of death.

Illness occurs whenever something disrupts the orderly functioning of the living system. We observe the breakdown of order and the damage to structures and functions in the symptoms which arise. In Chinese Medicine, factors which could potentially cause malfunction, disorder and disease were referred to as 'evil' because of the harm which they caused. On evil, the *Practical Dictionary of Chinese Medicine* defines it as: "Any entity from outside or from within that threatens health."[1]

Things which cause physiological disorder can be thought of thermodynamically as entropy-increasers. As Erwin Schrodinger pointed out in his book 'What is Life', a feature of living organisms is to maintain a state of thermodynamic non-equilibrium in the face of the second law of thermodynamics.

"Life seems to be orderly and lawful behaviour of matter, not based exclusively on its tendency to go over from order to disorder, but based partly on existing order that is kept up."
Erwin Schrödinger, What is Life?

In Chinese Medicine terms, the maintenance of this order is the function of the Zheng Qi; the righteous and upright nature of the body to maintain its own integrity and continue its optimal energetic functionalities. All of the healthy process of our body work in harmony to maintain this order and stability.

Imagine the body as a thermodynamic system where Zheng Qi is the natural physiological regulatory functions working to keep entropy stable by maintaining order out of complexity and maximizing efficient energy metabolism. Xie Qi endlessly introduces variables that challenge this regulation, pushing the system towards disorder and thus higher entropy. This results in inflammatory responses and the manifestation of symptoms depending upon how and where the system suffers disruption. Health then becomes a dynamic where Zheng Qi must continually adapt and respond to these challenges to restore or maintain order.

> *"'Evil' stands in opposition to the 'right', the force that maintains health."*
> *Practical Dictionary of Chinese Medicine*

A main goal of acupuncture is to support the adaptive upright Zheng Qi of the organism to sustain and reestablish harmony. One of the main ways to accomplish this is to defeat and drive out oppositional evils which threaten disruption and harm wherever they are found. Another way to do this is to support the inner coherency and strength of the structures and functions of the organism itself. In this sense, acupuncture can be thought of as metaphorically similar to the driving out of invaders, thieves, robbers, marauders or bandits terrorizing the inner economy of the empire.

---

1. A Practical Dictionary of Chinese Medicine

Yīn and Yáng

陰陽

Yin and Yang are the archetypical, primordial opposites hardcoded into the cosmology of nature. Everything can be understood according to the relativity of Yin and Yang. From a cosmological perspective, Yin is the solid earth below us while Yang is the airy skies above. Life occurs when novel forms emerge through the harmonious blending of Yin and Yang.

> *"Water is yin; fire is yang. Yang is Qi; Yin is flavor."*
> *Su Wen, Chapter 5*

The heat and movement of Yang is like fire, while the cool stillness of Yin is like water. Qi and function is the Yang to Yin's of Blood and structure. Yin and Yang can be applied to all phenomena, allowing us to understand the state of their relative balance on a spectrum.

> *"Yang Qi provides the [myriad beings] with proper Qi; Yin Qi rules them."*
> *Su Wen, Chapter 6*

The principle of Yin and Yang has fractal dimensions to it. There is another Yin and Yang nested within each Yin and Yang. This property allows deep observational and descriptive capabilities which can be applied to medicine and physiology and complex living systems. It is the basis of diagnostics as well as treatment.

> *"The Yang, that is the Qi of Heaven. It rules the outside. The Yin, that is the Qi of Earth. It rules the inside. Hence, the Yang paths are subject to repletion; the Yin paths are subject to depletion. Hence, when one is invaded*

by a robber wind or a depletion evil, the Yang conduits receive it. When food and drinks are consumed without restraint, when rising and resting occur out of time, the Yin conduits receive it. When the Yang conduits receive it, then it enters the six palaces. When the Yin conduits receive it, then it enters the five depots."
Su Wen, Chapter 29

Yin and Yang are not separate substances or forces. They are the two fundamental, reciprocal modes into which the undifferentiated unity of life divides. The terms originally referred to the shaded and sunny sides of a mountain slope, but the mountain itself remains one thing. Everything in existence can be observed through the lens of Yin and Yang's ceaseless transformations. Through Yin-Yang cosmology, we can locate where any phenomenon or process sits on this gradient within its ongoing cycle of change, read its propensities, anticipate its trajectory, and determine how best to act, applying acupuncture to intervene with maximum effect.

"One should take care to become familiar with Yin and Yang and one must not develop therapeutic schemes in the same way as ordinary practitioners."
Su Wen, Chapter 7

This quote warns us not to get caught in reflexive treatment patterns or unconscious habits which take away from one's ability to treat the actual context in front of them. The ability to step outside of therapeutic schemes requires spontaneity, intuition, and the willingness to follow the trail where it takes us, as opposed to trying to fit the situation into premeditated, artificial reasoning. In diagnosis, we must use Yin and Yang to understand the nature of the disharmony. Medicine then is the way to alter and shift the state of an organism back into a dynamic homeostasis. The purpose of acupuncture is to stimulate the Qi in such a way that this harmony is re-established naturally.

"The pattern of restoring harmony among the Qi must be tied to the Yin and Yang."
Nan Jing, Chapter 72

Heat and Cold

Heat and cold are a fundamental manifestation of Yin and Yang in our universe. As thermodynamics beings, we are extremely sensitive to the fluctuations of temperature and our bodies react and respond accordingly. We are also made primarily of water, which undergoes spontaneous phase changes if exposed to different temperatures. If a thermal imbalance occurs, this will disrupt the effectiveness of our physiological functions on a cellular and molecular level, and ultimately it can cause pain, symptoms and illness.

> *"The flow in the conduit vessels does not stop. It circulates without break. When cold Qi enters the conduits, stoppage and retardation result. The contents of the vessels are impeded to the degree that they fail to flow. When the cold Qi settles outside the vessels, then the blood is diminished [due to contraction / loss of flow]. When it settles inside the vessels, then the Qi cannot pass through. Hence, there is sudden pain."*
> *Su Wen, Chapter 39*

When there is cold in the conduits it causes pain. The blood congeals, circulation slows, and blocks can form. Moxibustion can be used to infuse warmth and Yang Qi to acupuncture points and unblock the constricting cold causing pain. Acupuncture helps to clear and open the channels.

Thermal imbalances often occur from the external environment. When external pathogens first strike the body they attack the exterior Yang portion. If left untreated, they can then progress internally, eventually reaching the organs. If a pathogen is still at the exterior and has not progressed beyond the conduits, venting the exterior and promoting sweating can help to clear it.

"When all three Yang conduits and network vessels have received this disease, and before it has entered the depots, one can make the patient sweat and the disease ends."
Su Wen, Chapter 31

Chapters 31 and 32 of the *Su Wen* are dedicated to the treatment of heat diseases with acupuncture. It is said that heat disorders can often cause severe mental emotional disturbances and manic, erratic behaviors. Heat diseases can manifest with different symptoms depending upon which organ is affected. Some useful acupuncture points below the vertebrae are specifically mentioned in Chapter 32 the *Su Wen* as 'heat Qi holes':

Below the 3rd vertebra → chest heat
Below the 4th vertebra → diaphragm heat
Below the 5th vertebrae → Liver heat
Below the 6th vertebrae → Spleen heat
Below the 7th vertebrae → Kidney heat

"The upper seven vertebrae are the Yang section; hence, they rule heat diseases."
Wu Kun, Su Wen Chapter 32 Commentary

Some of my favorite points for heat include LI11, LU5, SJ5, ST44, and HT8. Treat excessive heat by draining, cooling, discharging it; treat excessive cold by supplementing, warming and scattering it. Heat and cold can also be a result of internal imbalances of Yin and Yang. The classic describes heat diseases for every organ of the body. A common manifestation is when a patient suffering from Yin deficiency experiences heat, in which case SP6 and KD6 become operational points.

"The Yin Qi is diminished and the Yang Qi dominates. Hence, the body is hot, and the patient experiences vexation and fullness."
Su Wen, Chapter 34

Ultimately, we should strive for harmony in Yin and Yang and in the thermal regulation of heat and cold. This means engaging with the external environment appropriately, avoiding extreme weather conditions, and harmonizing with the seasons. Internally, this also means eating and drinking appropriately and moderating our behaviors. Choosing foods and beverages which harmonize our Qi and changing our diet with the seasons as necessary to the natural cycles of the year. Every food has an energetic quality to it, and excessive consumption of certain flavors can create imbalances over long periods of time. If our Zheng Qi is harmonious and strong we will be less susceptible to thermal fluctuations and external pathogens.

> *When piercing heat, wait for the arrival of cold, one must retain the needle; when Yīn Qì abundantly arrives, then exhale, remove it slowly, leaving their acupoint open and unobstructed. When piercing cold, wait for the arrival of heat; when Yáng Qì abundantly arrives, the needle's Qì must warm up, then inhale, remove it quickly, urgently pressing upon their acupoint.*
> *The Ode of Mysterious Indications, from the Zhenjiu Dacheng*

Blood

Xuè 血

Blood, the 'juice of life', is the essential substance that floods every fractal corner of our bodies with nourishment, sustaining cells and organs in a ceaseless flow. Every corner of the empire is provided with nutrients and life-giving vitality.

> *"The Qi is responsible for providing the body with a warm flow; the Blood is responsible for providing the body with moisture."*
> *Nan Jing, Chapter 22*

Without fresh blood we would dry up and die. Bodily structures will not be able to renew themselves with fertile Qi. Cells, tissues, and organs, would eventually break down and accumulate stagnancy, becoming like dead, lifeless, hardened soil where water does not reach and nothing grows. The ongoing autopoetic feedback loop of self-reconstruction and nourishment is critical to longevity, health and life. Hua Shou's commentary speaks to the importance of blood for the nourishment of the body:

> *"The Blood is responsible for providing the body with moisture' means that man's blood vessels moisten his muscles and bones, soften his joints, and nourish his organs."*
> *Hua Shou, Nan Jing Chapter 22 Commentary*

Blood is a primordial form, the Yin correlate to Yang's Qi. Like Yin and Yang, Qi and blood are inseparable; two parts to a whole. A famous principle encapsulates this interdependence:

"Qi is the commander of Blood, Blood is the mother of Qi."
TCM Principle

When we perform acupuncture we are working with the Qi and by extension the blood. Supplementing the Qi can supplement the production of blood, and vice versa. Some of my favorite points for supplementing the blood include: BL17, SP6 and SP10 as core blood-building points. ST36 and CV6 to nourish the blood by supplementing the Qi. BL18 and LV8 by supporting the Liver, which has the function of governing the blood. Or BL23, CV4, and KD3 to strengthen the Kidneys, thereby benefitting blood production by supporting the Jing essence and the marrow.

Each of the Jingmai channels are known to have differing proportions of Qi and Blood. Understanding these differences can also guide our point selection. Chapter 24 of the *Su Wen* overviews this topic:

Jingmai Qi and blood proportions:
Taiyang → much Qi, little blood
Shaoyang → little blood, much Qi
Yangming → much Qi, much blood
Shaoyin → little blood, much Qi
Jueyin → much blood, little Qi
Taiyin → much Qi, little blood

Where there is much blood, and it has stagnated to excess, it is appropriate to use bloodletting. We should not forget that blood letting is an essential part of needling and of acupuncture practice. *The Manual of Acupuncture* states that, "disorders of blood may be generalized as being of three main types: blood stasis, blood heat and blood deficiency."[1]

"When one has been struck by evil, one must attack the evil. However, the treatment should be early and one must quickly have the evil leave, thereby removing overly abundant blood. As a result, the Zheng Qi will return by itself. This way, in the draining there is also supplementation."
Zhang Jeibin

The primary therapeutic objective of bloodletting is to release malign blood, often seen as dark, stagnant, toxic blood stasis within the superficial vessels and collaterals. Draining this stagnant blood ensures that bad blood is cleared before it can penetrate into the deep channels to generate more severe visceral diseases. Typically, the malign blood first emerges as black, purple, or dark-colored, and the acupuncturist halts the treatment as soon as the blood turns to a normal, healthy red color. This change symbolizes the juice of life returning to a state of harmony.

---

1. Manual of Acupuncture

Structure and Function

"'Form follows function' is mere dogma until you realize the higher truth that form and function are one."
Frank Lloyd Wright

Structure and function are two inseparable sides to the same coin, like Yin and Yang. They are integral, ubiquitous aspects of biology and physiology and the evolutionary development of this self-organizing phenomenon we call life.[1]

The ancients understood Qi and form as one. Structure shapes function; while function defines structure. Each facilitates the other's expression and constrains one another's possibilities.

As our physiological state changes through time and with age, so do all of our physiological structures, as well as their functional efficiency. States of health and disease, harmony and disorder, are thus inevitably reflected through both the structures and the functions of the living organism. Whenever there is disease or disorder, we will find a disruption in function coinciding with a corresponding degradation to physiological structures.

Yin and Yang embody this principle in the most archetypal sense. Yin represents the structural, dense, material, substantial aspects of life while Yang represents its functional, energetic, active, operative qualities. Therefore, each thing in the universe contains an interdependently intertwined Yin structure and Yang function. This duality can be seen in the relationship between Blood and Qi in acupuncture theory – they are physiological archetypes of structure and function.

Ultimately, these two polarities are intimately and inseparably linked. When an organism is in a state of health, its structures can be seen to conform to their proper shape, size, or color. When it is in a state of disease, we can clearly see the disorganization as deformations, discolorations, and visual signs of a breakdown of normalcy. This is a fundamental aspect of diagnosis. The state of various structures implies the corresponding functional capacities of an organism. Conversely, if we begin to observe the breakdown of a function, we may intuit that its corresponding structural integrity is compromised. If the Qi is disordered, we may expect the problem to also affect the Blood, and vice versa.

When structures and functions deteriorate, this results in thermodynamic inefficiencies, increased entropy, disrupted communication and information flows, and the energy availability of the system is reduced by the inherent disorganization and chaos — in other words, disease. Integrity of structure and function is the property of upright, proper Zheng Qi, and is therefore synonymous with health.

Alternatively, when structures and functions become pathologically rigid or overly constrained, the system loses the variability and dynamical complexity required for adaptation. Communication and information flows grow stereotyped and inflexible, free energy becomes trapped in fixed patterns rather than being flexibly redeployed, and the organism can no longer explore the range of potential states needed to meet changing demands. The result is a loss of resilience and responsiveness — in other words, disease of a different kind, driven not by rising disorder but by excessive, constraining order.

Acupuncture stimulation uses strategic perturbations in order to direct the body's attention to the fractal holographic aspect of disruption. This engages the systemic healing response so that the body can muster its resources — both defensive and constructive — in order to regulate and re-establish a harmonious state of Qi by expelling pathogens, repairing and maintaining structures, and re-optimizing their proper functions.

---

1. The Structure and Function of Living Organisms

Essence

Jīng 精

Jing, or essence, is fundamentally one's potential at any given movement. Etymologically, the Chinese character for Jing represents a pure, fine grain of uncooked rice. Jing is "the unadulterated essence of things or a state of mind that is concentrated on a single purpose. It is also used to refer to the seed of human life."[1] Therefore, it is also commonly equated with seminal essence, which is physiologically symbolic of the ultimate potential for creating a human life.

We inherit our Jing, or congenital essence, from our parents at the moment of conception, and through the process of gestation and birth. It is not uncommon to find similarities between Jing and genetics, or even stem cells.[2] Jing is one's vitality and constitution, one's most refined, essential nature. Essence can therefore be partly understood as one's fated allotment of potential by the universe.

> *"Two spirits communicate and combine to give birth to form. What existed prior to the birth of the body is called essence."*
> *Ling Shu, Chapter 30*

In terms of nature versus nurture, Jing refers to one's inborn nature. This is sometimes referred to as 'earlier heaven essence'. But potential must also be nurtured. The nourishment and cultivation of one's potential during life can be understood as 'later heaven essence'.[3] Our actions either preserve and cultivate our Jing, or they spend it, or even waste it. This is part of the basis of the tradition of Nourishing Life, Yang Sheng. To manifest our utmost potential requires nature as well as nurture.

At any moment a variety of unique possibilities and potentials, flowing from our inherited Jing, our accumulated choices, and current position, are available to each individual. We can call these possibilities '*adjacent possibles*'. When we are in a state of health and our spirits are bright, our unique potentials and possibilities are expansive and vast. What we can be, what we can do, or where we can go — a panoply of possibilities exist adjacent to who, what, and where one is right now. One job of the acupuncturist is to help inform, advise, and nourish every patient to the best of our abilities in order to maximize and unfold these adjacent possibles towards their highest ideal and purpose. When we nourish our potential and fulfill its promise, we manifest our destiny for the benefit of the self, the community, and society at large.

> *"One must value the essence. When the essence is plentiful, the Qi becomes exuberant. When Qi is exuberant, the spirit is sound. When the spirit is sound, the physique is strong. And when the physique is strong, there is less disease."*
> *Leijing, Volume One*

Disruptions to our Qi can potentially harm our Jing. When we become ill or injured, the possibilities available to us shrinks. We cannot manifest our greatest purpose while we fight off pathogens or heal disharmonies afflicting our Zhong Qi. Or if an injury is keeping us from doing the things we love or are meant to do in life. A premature death is a tragic end to potential and an extinguishing of essence.

Before acupuncture, a patient's condition might be such that there is a high likelihood of them continuing to be sick or injured, or perhaps it may even worsen. This constricts what is possible for them. We use acupuncture to shift the adjacent possibles of a sick patient towards a higher probability of health – a nudge towards a new homeodynamic harmony where Qi flows optimally again.

Acupuncture can thus be seen as an event that changes the transition probabilities between states. Through treatment, we can help to rescue and restore the essence of the patient by intervening and expanding the adjacent potentials available to them.

---

1. Guanzi: Political, Economic, and Philosophical Essays from Early China

2. Shen-Jing as a Chinese Medicine Concept Might Be a Counterpart of Stem Cells in Regenerative Medicine

3. A Practical Dictionary of Chinese Medicine

Living Points

Not every point on the body will be effective or optimal for treatment, so we seek the most impactful areas within the context of each situation. Diagnosing the sick channel is the first step in the process. Then we apply reason and theory to choose the relevant treatment zones so that we can locate effective acupuncture points. If we want to be most effective, we must focus and zoom in to find the specific spots which will actually be needled. Honing in further and becoming even more accurate and exacting with our needle placement will get us even closer to the best results. We want to find the most potent Qi holes, and accurately.

Shudō Denmei describes this as a process of finding 'living points'.[1] The process of finding the most active acupuncture points on an acupuncture channel is achieved by using our palpation skills. Learning to use our hands and developing our sense of touch is one of the most important skills we can have as acupuncturists.

Active, living points, will identify themselves to us through palpation. Sometimes they present themselves as ashi points, so we must verbally communicate with patients to get their feedback. Since much of communication is nonverbal, we must also attentively observe their involuntary and spontaneous bodily reactions and body language.

We may feel living points as areas of abnormality under our fingers during palpation. They can feel like emptiness or a fullness, a hardness or a softness, as rough or lumpy tissues, or as tight and stagnant tissues, for example. We must learn to use our senses to their fullest in order to find the most accurate points possible.

If we find a living point, we can use it as a central point in a Dao Ma configuration and apply appropriate techniques for supplementation or drainage.

---

1. Finding Effective Acupuncture Points

Mutuality of Opposites

Acupuncture requires us to understand and influence Yin and Yang. Yin and Yang are at the foundation of both diagnosis and treatment. This is because these are the primordial forces of the universe. Archetypically, they are understood to represent Heaven and Earth, light and dark, formless ethereality and dense substance. By virtue of this, health, illness, and medicine are dependent upon them. All things are composed of them and all changes occur through their interactions. Understanding this, we can apply acupuncture in order to effect a change and initiate a movement towards a greater harmony.

> *"Those who know how to use the needles, from the yin they pull the yang and from the yang they pull the yin. With the right they treat the left and with the left they treat the right. From this they know that; from the exterior they know the interior. By observing the structures of excess and inadequacy, they see the minute and notice the excess. When they apply the needles, there will be no failure."*
> *Su Wen, Chapter 5*

For this reason, it is not uncommon to use opposite aspects of the body in treatment. For diseases above, we can treat them from below. For diseases below, we can treat them from above. In the *Ling Shu*, this is called 'Needling the Distant Road'.

> *"If the disease is located in the upper body, treat the lower body. If the disease is located in the lower part, treat the upper. If the disease is located in the head, treat the feet. If disease is located in the loins, treat the crease of the knee."*
> *Ling Shu, Chapter 9*

Similarly, we can treat diseases on the right from the left, and diseases on the left from the right. In the *Ling Shu*, this is referred to as 'Opposite Needling.' It is also sometimes referred to as a 'Misleading Piercing'.

> *"In piercing the network vessels, if evil is on the left, take it from the right; if it is on the right, take it from the left."*
> *Wang Bing*

The body is a unified fractal whole. The unity of opposites, Yin and Yang is the archetype of this. Understanding the complete unity and interconnectedness, it is a natural conclusion that opposites can treat each other. If we pull one end of a thread, it will move the opposite end as well. In fact, this is a guiding principle for how we see the natural world and the human body.

> *"Man is that which makes a triad with heaven and earth and has resonances with yin and yang."*
> *Ling Shu, Chapter 79*[1]

---

1. See also, Su Wen Chapter 25.

What is the Point?

Only put a needle somewhere if it has a purpose. Don't place needles without a clear goal or a predetermined strategy in mind. Always have a reason for doing something. Experimentation and creativity are okay, that is part of the process of learning. But even experiments must have a hypothesis and a logical theory behind them. If we find ourselves doing things without a rational basis which we can clearly explain, it is time to slow down, center, and simplify, starting from first principles.

> *"As a general principle, there must be a reason why a thing is as it is. If you do not understand that reason, then whether what you do is appropriate to the circumstances or not, the end result is the same: you are certain to encounter problems. The way in which ancient kings, famous scholar-knights, and accomplished teachers surpassed the ordinary people of their age was in knowing the reasons. Rivers do not flow out of mountains and rush to the sea because they have an aversion to mountains and love the sea."*
> *The Annals of Lü Buwei, Book 9 Chapter 4.1*

It is important to put in the time, to do the learning, to build and gather experience, so that there is a theoretical basis for everything that we do. Even if we hit our target, if we do not know how we did so then we have more work to do in order to understand the reasons behind things. Our patients are depending upon us to make good choices and sound decisions based on reason and logic with our treatment strategies. This means that acupuncture and medicine, like war, benefits from an ongoing process of preparation, study, experience, and work. One of the best ways to build experience is to treat as many patients as possible. The process continues in silence, in the time spent studying, reading, thinking about the art. This preparation pre-configured builds the propensity for victory, like the gathering of momentum and gravity. Victory occurs long before the patient walks into the clinic.

> *"Thus it is that in war the victorious strategist only seeks battle after the victory has been won, whereas he who is destined to defeat first fights and afterwards looks for victory."*
> *Sunzi, Chapter 4.15*

Acupuncture is a very gentle, safe, forgiving, and effective medical practice. But the classics make it clear that if it is not performed properly, it can also cause harm and make matters worse. Our first principle is to do no harm. The easiest way to make a disease worse is to do something which does not have a clear and rational basis behind it. The best way to ensure a logical approach to a treatment is to do the work beforehand. Understand the principles, theories, and methods, so that each thing we do is imbued with the most intention possible for the highest chance of effectiveness and positive outcomes.

Propensity

Shì 勢

One of the most pivotal concepts in Chinese philosophy is *shì*, which can be understood as the propensity at work in reality. Everything has a certain propensity, and this is based on its configuration among the dynamic state of reality. Just as water has its tendency to flow downwards as gravity exerts its force upon the world, everything has a certain propensity towards where it is going and how it is going to end up. To go against the propensity of things is absurd and leads to disaster. Shì is like the energy of a loaded, drawn crossbow. This potential can and will be unleashed, so use it effectively, but don't get in its way. This is why the sages sought to behave according to the principles of reality, and their actions harmonized with the tendencies of nature.

> *"The Way engenders them,*
> *Virtue nurtures them,*
> *Material reality confers physical form on them,*
> *And propensity brings them to full fruition."*
> *Dao De Jing, Chapter 51*

Human beings are subject to the propensity at work in reality. We are all born with an allotment of essence and potential which can unfold in many directions. Our habits and practices build up over time and yield inevitable results, like the momentum of rocks dislodged to then roll down from the top of a mountain. Just as there is an art of warfare, there is also an art to living, to nourishing one's life, to practicing acupuncture, and whatever else is aspired to. The ancient sages sought "to act in a way to ensure one's victory, by making it predetermined. Ultimately, every ideal outcome depends 'simply' on getting the operative and controlling effect in any given situation to work towards its achievement."[1] Part of our job as acupuncturists is to assess the state of a patient's Qi, the configuration of Yin and Yang, and determine the changes and transformations needed to bring harmony and health back to the system and to achieve a medical victory. We can help them correct habits and practices which lead to an assuredly negative future conclusion, and we can intervene strategically with acupuncture to shift the tides of a current battle. By reconfiguring the situation, we can change the propensity of reality to deliver a positive result. But it is easier to change the outcome before it builds up steam; catch it when it is just a tiny sprout and pluck it like a weed. Unfortunately, many patients will reach us when their issue is a boulder barreling down a mountain with extreme velocity and force.

> *"Since the beginnings of good and bad fortune are tiny as a sprout, people overlook them. Only sages see their beginnings and know their ends."*
> *Huainanzi, Chapter 10.24*

As acupuncturists, we also have our own propensity at work. We are like the general in many ways — the work we do before the moment of the battle determines the results. The successful general has already done the calculations and worked out the path to victory; has organized circumstances in such a way that the outcome is assured before the battle takes place. Similarly, the acupuncturist who achieves success in a myriad of cases has spent the time learning the subtle mechanisms of acupuncture. They have gathered experience, mastered the art of attaining the Qi, and are intimate with the channels and collaterals, the terrain, inner workings, and principles of the body – in short, they have assessed the details down to the finest autumn hair. Because they have spent their time in preparation, the acupuncture is performed in such a way that it perfectly exerts the required leverage to shift the current state of physiological reality and successful results flow from this effortlessly.

> *"Thus, the distinction between order and disorder, survival and destruction, when it is first manifest, is as subtle as autumn hair. If one examines large undertakings down to their 'autumn hairs', then they will not go off course."*
> *The Annals of Lü Buwei, Chapter 16/6.1*

---

1. The Propensity of Things: Towards a History of Efficacy in China.

Fractal Self-Similarity

The universe is a fractal, and so is the environment in which we live. We, too, as products of the universe and our environment, are ourselves fractal beings.[1] The ancients intuited this, and so they understood that the rivers, mountains, and other natural features of the world followed the same universal principles which also govern human physiology. They organized themselves accordingly, sought out the natural correspondences, and harmonized themselves with the natural rhythms of life.

Self-similarity means that when we zoom in and out of a fractal, the same picture presents itself. We can extrapolate the inner from the outer, we can understand what is above from what it is below. Left and right treat one another. Yin and Yang give birth to one another. The Yin Yang symbol is the archetypal representation of the fractal nature of reality. It is a network of systems within systems.

When we look at the topography of the landscape from above, we will see the fractal nature of the forms. The coastlines, the mountains, and the river basins. When we look closely at our bodies, we see similar organizational principles at work. Our brains and nervous systems, our circulatory systems and the complex network of capillaries, veins, and arteries, our lungs and the tree-like alveoli. Every aspect of our being is composed according to fractal principles. These sorts of structures lend themselves naturally to energy conservation and optimal organizational efficiency. When systems and organisms arrange themselves according to the most effective thermodynamic conditions, they become more adaptive and thrive amidst evolutionary competition and environmental constraints.

> *"Therefore, regarding the human body; then the exterior is the branch, the interior is the root; Yáng is the branch, Yīn is the root; the Yáng bowels are the branch, the Yīn viscera are the root; the viscera and bowels located interiorly are the root, the channels and collaterals located exteriorly are the branch."*
> *The Ode of Mysterious Indications, from the Zhenjiu Dacheng*

We take advantage of fractal reality in our diagnosis and acupuncture treatment. We observe microcosms to understand the macrocosm. We observe the exterior to understand the interior. The root and the branch are as one. When everything is an interconnected fractal whole, it is simple to see how an acupuncture needle can have a systemic effect. The acupuncture channels are mathematical contours following the fractal principles of the universe, but applied to the structure of our being.

---

1. The Fractal Tapestry of Life

Resonances

"If you want to find the secrets of the universe, think in terms of energy, frequency and vibration."
Nikola Tesla

The human body is a multi-fractal with features of self-similarity, and we can observe the whole through the parts. Just like when we look at fractal objects in nature, when we zoom in or out the objects once again appear to us as fractal self-similars at each of the various scales of magnification. Ultimately, the parts resonate with the frequency of the whole. This is the basis of many of the diagnostic techniques of acupuncture.

"Clouds are not spheres, mountains are not cones, coastlines are not circles, and bark is not smooth, nor does lightning travel in a straight line."
Benoit Mandelbrot

Rather than attempt to apply reductive, deterministic reasoning to a system as infinitely complex as the human physiological system, the diagnostic methods of acupuncture take a different route and use a different strategy. They seek to ascertain the resonant frequency, the overall qualitative energetic state of the system as a whole. In other words, the goal is to understand the Qi. The Qi is revealed through all aspects of the system's manifestation. The harmonics of Yin and Yang express themselves through the pulse, the tongue, the physical appearance, the sounds and language, the emotions, and the entire constellation of symptoms.

"Examine the external resonances of the body in order to know the body's viscera. Thus you will know what is diseased."
Ling Shu, Chapter 47

The diagnostic techniques of acupuncture give insight into the overall state of Qi. It reveals the resonant frequency of the system and points to the nature and origin of disharmony. The different pulse shapes, tongue patterns, colors, sounds, and symptoms, resonate in harmony with the overall tuning of the system at large. Only by understanding the nature of how a living system has become disharmonious can we hope to apply acupuncture in order to stimulate a return back to a state of harmony.

"Man's color and pulse are like measures and have mutual resonances, like a drumstick and a drum. The shape of the sounds are mutually resonating; without attainment, they are mutually lost. These relationships are like cause and effect, like the roots of the tree and the leaves which come out of it, for the death of the root causes the withered leaf. Color, pulse, form and flesh cannot be separated. To know one method is to possess technique, to know two methods is to possess Spirit, and to know three methods is to possess Spirit as well as Vision."
Ling Shu, Chapter 4

Images

Xiàng 象

"Men seldom see a living elephant. They obtain the skeleton of a dead elephant and imagine a living one according to its features. Whatever people use for imagining the real is called 'an elephant/an image' (xiang)."
Han Feizi

The character *xiang* originally meant, literally, 'elephant.' But as wild elephants grew scarce in the central plains of China during the Warring States period, philosophers repurposed the noun to describe how human consciousness reconstructs a reality it cannot directly observe. Over time, this concept evolved to mean an 'image' which functions as a sort of bridge between the metaphysical and the physical. The visible pattern reveals itself as an image through which an invisible, formless reality becomes accessible.

Applied to medicine, the state of Qi in a patient's system displays itself as a pattern; an image of the Qi. When we perform diagnostics on a patient, we are looking for outward signs which tell us about the inner condition. This image takes the form of the pulse, or the color of the face, or is heard in the quality of the voice. Perhaps the patient's prevailing emotions express the pattern of disharmony, or they give off a scent which hints at the prevailing state of Qi. What displays itself is the composite of the entire manifestation of the patient's Qi.

"The [movements in the] vessels, be they minor or strong, smooth or rough, at the surface or in the depth, they can be differentiated with the fingers. The images [of the conditions] of the five depots, they can be deduced through comparison. ... As for the examination of the subtle appearances of the five complexions, they can be inspected with the eyes. Those who are able to match the [movement in the] vessels and complexion, they can achieve myriad

cures."
Su Wen, Chapter 10

Each of these signs gives us clues about which organ system is in disharmony. We could see an abnormality in a specific tissue; this acts as a visible aspect of the image of the Qi of the patient. A physical abnormality in a specific tissue is therefore never merely local — problems with the sinews read as a Liver disorder, while skin or body-hair changes reveal a compromised Lung, and so on. The premise that the macrocosm and microcosm express one another means that the hidden internal state of the organs and the channels is constantly and faithfully projected onto the body's external surfaces as legible, dynamic images.

By learning the images of Qi, we are able to understand the underlying pattern and immediately recognize the meanings of the signs and symptoms which the patient displays. By performing acupuncture, we aim to directly intervene and change this pattern. The image of Qi is dynamic; it continually responds to whatever transformations occur.

"When the Qi ends, the images change."
Su Wen, Chapter 70

Diagnostics

"To examine and to know the Yin and Yang is to have the rules of acupuncture. When the beginning of the disease has been located, needling will have a foundation."
Ling Shu, Chapter 6

Before any treatment plan can be developed or any acupuncture treatment can take place, diagnostics must be performed and the disease must be located and understood. Without diagnosis, we are throwing darts with a blindfold on.

The human body is an extremely complex physiological system with a vast amount of processes, layers and dimensions all operating interconnectedly and simultaneously. Attempting to approach this level of complexity through a reductionist lens may be an impossible task. Rather than attempt this, we can view the classical acupuncture diagnostic methods instead as holographic snapshots of the entire fractal system.

"Complexion and movement of the vessels, this is what the Lords on High valued; the teachers of former times have transmitted it."
Su Wen, Chapter 13

Techniques such as taking the pulse of a patient or inspecting their tongue are used to approximate the current state of their highly complex system at that moment in time. We may not have the ability to measure every minute deterministic physiological detail in a linear reductionist way, but the genius of acupuncture diagnostic methods is that they take the different route of attempting to ascertain a probabilistic, pattern-based diagnosis.

> *"The complexion is that by which a physician establishes correspondences to the sun. The movement of the vessels is that by which a physician establishes correspondences to the moon."*
> *Su Wen, Chapter 13*

We can think of the pulse, the tongue, and complexion, and other diagnostic data, as observable stochastic samples of the patient's Qi. Just as in any fractal phenomenon which displays self-similarity at different scales, the patterns of the patient's Qi will reveal itself and be observable through the pulse pattern and various other manifestations. The ecosystem of the body will express itself through their tongue pattern and their complexion. In this way, it is like observing the Sun and the Moon of their inner universe.

> *"The most essential in treatment is the following: not to miss movement in the vessels and complexion, and to make use of them without confusion, that is the grand rule of treatment."*
> *Su Wen, Chapter 13*

The Pulse

"The movement in the vessels is most decisive for man."
Chang Shih-hsien, Nan Jing Chapter 21 Commentary

The pulse is the gateway to the inner energetic resonance of the human body. The ancients knew that the pulse is like a mirror to the Qi of the patient. If there is disease, it will be reflected in the quality and pattern of the pulse.

"Anybody who feels the vessels and knows it is to be called a skilled workman."
Nan Jing, Chapter 61

Part of the art of pulse taking is understanding the patterns of the pulse and the inner Qi states which they reflect and represent. Yin and Yang reflect themselves differently. Deep or shallow, front or back, hot or cold; the Qi will express itself on the pulse according to the prevailing state of the overall system. The best way to learn the nuances of pulse diagnosis is to feel as many pulses as possible. Read the classics to gain the experience of the doctors and masters who laid the foundation of the art and utilize their insights.

"The movements in the vessels be they minor or big, smooth or rough, at the surface or in the depth, they can be differentiated with the fingers."
Su Wen, Chapter 10

Stochastic observables are quantities or measurements within a stochastic (random or probabilistic) process or system which can be observed or measured. Pulse taking reveals both quantifiable and qualitative data to the practitioner about the state and nature of the patient's fractal holistic processes and system. In short, it reveals the overall state of their Qi. It is like sensing the sound waves of a piece of music - the emotional undertones and qualities of the piece reveal themselves naturally if we are sensitive and observant.

> *"Those who are able to match the movement in the vessels and complexion, they can achieve success in a myriad of cases."*
> *Su Wen, Chapter 10*

Fractal behavior in living beings is the norm rather than the exception, and fractal dynamics in the behaviors of complex networks such as living systems is ubiquitous.[1] The heartbeat as well as the breath both have characteristics of fractal time series and stochastic processes. In other words, they display self-similar patterns at different scales and time lengths, as well as contain considerable variability and also inherent randomness. The cardiovascular system and the lungs are both prime examples of physiological structures with fractal geometries. The reason the pulse can reflect so much is precisely *because* it's a fractal, self-similar signal, so reading it well is a skill to be practiced, learned, and developed over a life time.

---

1. The Fractal Tapestry of Life

The Tongue

The physiology of an organism is like a whole ecosystem. Just as planet earth contains various continents, mountain ranges and oceans, the human body is a self-contained system with ecological diversity. Some areas should be wet, others should be dry, just as some can run colder while others can run hotter.

When ecosystems go out of balance, there can be collapse of the feedback systems which sustain it. The health of the entire ecosystem is in a holistic, integrated relationship with itself. If an area goes through a drought or a cold snap, or if a natural disaster like a fire rages through the landscape, it can devastate the entire ecosystem. That being said, ecosystems are fairly resilient structures which can survive intense events like these and recover. Similarly, the human body is also incredibly resilient and capable of repair and harmonization.

One way to gain a view into the ecosystem of the body is through tongue diagnosis, which is part of the art of visual inspection. When we look at the tongue of a patient we gain a glimpse into a microcosmic representation of the entire state of their physiological bodily ecology. Any disturbances in the harmony of their inner ecosystems will be represented on the tongue.

> *"Following the principle that "the part reflects the whole", localized signs such as tongue characteristics and pulse conditions are considered micro-projections of the body's overall Qi, blood, Yin, and Yang status."*[1]

If a patient is dry, their tongue will look dry and will lack a coating. If a patient is hot, their tongue will be red and the coat may turn yellow, reflecting the heat. If a patient is damp, their tongue will be swollen, as if filled with fluids. All of the many various visual signs of tongue diagnosis reflect an actual ecological state within some part of the patient. We can tell if the ecological situation underlying the disease resembles that of a desert, a marsh, a tundra, or a blazing fire. These examples of extreme ecological conditions which are difficult for life to thrive in are metaphors for states of disharmony and imbalance which can manifest in the body, disrupting normal functioning and causing symptoms of disease and disorder.

Tongue diagnosis enables us to understand the bodily ecology so that we can restore order and harmonize the inner environment, much like a terraforming process. If a patient is dry, moisten them. If a patient is cold, warm them. Dry the swamps and cleanse the phlegm; cool the blazing heat and douse the fires. Reduce excesses and nourish deficiencies. For this, we use acupuncture and also herbal medicines.

---

1. Foundation and Practice of Digital Traditional Chinese Medicine Platforms in Enhanced Recovery After Surgery

Holographics

Since the human body is a fractal structure with self-similar properties, each part can be used as a holographic representation of other aspects or even the whole. There are microcosms and macrocosms, worlds within worlds, and this can be used to our advantage during diagnosis and also treatment. Because of this holographic and self-similar design, every local part reflects the information of the whole, allowing a microscopic stimulus to instantaneously cascade throughout the global biological network.

This is why diagnostics such as the pulse and tongue can be used to approximate the entire holistic state of the organism. They are minimaps for the entire system. There are multitudes of ways in which the whole represents itself within creative holographic microcosms. The ears, the palms, the feet; these are prime examples of microcosmic holograms applied for this purpose. But really, any part of the body can be used creatively to create a distal holographic relationship. Because the whole is reflected in its individual parts, a practitioner can strategically use a distal point on a limb to treat a diseased area elsewhere.

In Master Tung's system, holographic correspondences are scaled into three distinct sizes, allowing the practitioner to project the diseased area onto different distal zones of the body.

- Large Taiji: This maps parts of the body that are of similar size and proportion.
  - Limb-to-Limb: A diseased extremity is projected onto its opposite counterpart. For example, the left hand treats the right foot, the shoulder treats the contralateral hip, and the elbow treats the contralateral knee. It can also be inverted, meaning the hand treats the contralateral shoulder.
  - Trunk-to-Limb: The entire trunk and head are mapped onto the entire arm or leg. In a normal orientation, the head corresponds to the hand/foot, the navel/waist corresponds to the elbow/knee, and the genital area corresponds

to the shoulder/hip.

- Medium Taiji: This maps the entire trunk and head only onto the lower portions of the extremities (distal to the knees or elbows). In this smaller hologram, the wrist and ankle represent the waist/navel area, the fingers/toes represent the head, and the areas closer to the elbow/knee represent the genital regions.

- Small Taiji: This maps the entire body onto comparatively small areas, such as a single tubular bone (like a metacarpal or the tibia), the sole of the foot, or the head. For example, the shaft of a single long bone can be divided into segments corresponding to the head, thorax, abdomen, and pelvis.

The relationship between Taiji as the universal macrocosm and the individual parts (microcosms) of the world is not one of a whole broken into fractions. Instead, it perfectly describes what we would call a holographic or fractal reality, where the entirety of the whole is fully present within every single part.

Dr. Tan structured his distal point selection into two specific formats that echo Master Tung's Taiji concepts:

1. The Mirroring Format (Limb-to-Limb) The Mirroring Format creates a direct map between the upper limbs and lower limbs.

- Standard Mirror: The finger mirrors the toe, the wrist mirrors the ankle, the elbow mirrors the knee, and the shoulder mirrors the hip.

- Reverse Mirror: By inverting the map, the finger mirrors the top of the hip, the wrist mirrors the hip joint, the elbow mirrors the knee, and the shoulder mirrors the ankle. This allows a practitioner to treat shoulder joint pain by needling the ankle, maximizing patient comfort.

2. The Imaging Format (Limb-to-Body) The Imaging Format relates a single limb to the entire head and trunk. Dr. Tan noted that any boney section of the body (including the ears, hands, feet, and scalp) can serve as a microcosm to image the entire body.

- Standard Image: The hand images the head, the wrist images the neck, the forearm images the chest, the elbow crease images the navel, and the shoulder images the groin and sacrum.

- Reverse Image: When the image is inverted, the hand/fingers image the genital and groin region, the elbow still images the navel, the upper arm images the chest, and the shoulder images the head. Thus, genital pain can easily be treated by needling the hand or the foot.

- Scalp Imaging: The midline of the scalp can also image the spine, allowing scalp points to treat problems along the posterior or anterior aspects of the body.

To successfully utilize these holographic connections, one does not simply needle a generalized area. After determining the correct holographic map, the practitioner firmly palpates the distal area to find an "ashi" point. The presence of this tender spot confirms the holographic connection between the distal limb and the sick meridian, making it the exact location to insert the needle to achieve instantaneous relief.

Channel Relationships

"All matter, which has form, has a geometric pattern which describes this form. Matter, which grows in a systematic and regular array of patterns, is spoken of as crystalline."
Marcel Vogel

The Jingluo theory of the channels originates from universal principles. It is a mathematical system for understanding the planes of the liquid-crystalline body. Our bodies are liquid-crystalline by their nature; primarily composed of water. Our connective tissues and fascia are built from collagen, which is likewise crystalline. Like a crystal, we form according to geometric and mathematical principles. These are made evident by the naturally forming relationships which occur between the planes of the body. Channel mathematics has its roots in the basic binary relationship of Yin and Yang.

"All the major constituents of living organisms, from lipids of cellular membranes to DNA, possibly all proteins, especially cytoskeletal proteins, muscle proteins, and proteins in the connective tissues such as collagens and proteoglycans, may be liquid crystalline."[1]

The channels develop and exist in a crystalline array configured in relation to one another. Once we understand these relationships it becomes easy to see how acupuncture can 'touch and influence' one part of the physiological universe from opposite or corresponding parts. We can touch the bottom from the top, the left from the right, the inside from the outside; mathematical relationships exist in many forms. This means there are many different ways by which we can access and influence any sick channel with acupuncture. This is epitomized in the five systems of channel relationships used by Dr. Tan. These systems give us an effective means to tap into the crystalline nature of our physiology. This idea gives a deeper meaning to acupuncture: it does not simply pierce, it taps into a fractal crystalline geometry. To needle one point and feel its effect resolve in a distant plane of the body is only strange if we forget that we are, ourselves, crystalline — patterned matter, arranged in relationship, all the way down.

---

1. Deep into the Water: Exploring the Hydro-Electromagnetic and Quantum Electrodynamic Properties of Interfacial Water in Living Systems.

Crystal Plane Mirroring

Imagine the body as a collection of crystalline planes in mathematical relationship to one another. A multifaceted, liquid-crystalline structure. The structure contains a front and a back plane, a medial and lateral plane, and an intermediate plane. Symbolically, these six channels are organized using an architectural metaphor of a door to represent their energetic functions in managing the flow of Qi between the exterior and interior.

> *"In the division and unity of the three Yang vessels, the Tai Yang is the opening; the Yang Ming is the door leaf; the Shao Yang is the pivot. In the division and unity of the three Yin vessels, the Tai Yin is the opening; the Jue Yin is the door leaf; the Shao Yin is the pivot."*
> *Su Wen, Chapter 6*

The geometric, crystalline nature of the body reflects the principle by which it developed, its structure follows this principle. This is why we can tap into the relationship between them in a geometric, mathematical way. This is the fundamental insight of Dr. Tan's five systems, which tap into the cosmological holographic principle at the foundation of Chinese philosophy. These systems rely on the symmetry of channel nomenclature, organ pairings, and the cyclical geometry of the Chinese clock. The systems function as the relational crystalline matrix of the channels, and they give us a precise method to take practical, directed actions upon any diseased channels.

System 1 (Chinese Meridian Name-Sharing): This creates a direct 1:1 correlation between hand and foot channels that share the exact same Chinese name. For example, the Hand *Tai Yin* (Lung) is balanced by the Foot *Tai Yin* (Spleen).

System 2 (Branching Meridians): This system balances channels based on the mutual attraction of specific paired names. Hand and foot channels are cross-paired in a strict pattern: *Tai Yin* balances *Tai Yang*, *Shao Yin* balances *Shao Yang*, and *Jue Yin* balances *Yang Ming*.

System 3 (Interior/Exterior Pairs): This system balances the traditional *Zang-Fu* (solid and hollow organ) pairs. It is the only system where a hand channel directly balances another hand channel, and a foot balances a foot (e.g., Foot *Jue Yin* Liver balances Foot *Shao Yang* Gallbladder).

System 4 (Chinese Clock Opposites): This system utilizes the circular geometry of the 12-hour Chinese clock. Meridians that sit exactly 12 hours apart on opposite sides of the clock balance each other (e.g., Foot *Tai Yin* Spleen at 9-11 a.m. is balanced by Hand *Shao Yang* San Jiao at 9-11 p.m.).

System 5 (Chinese Clock Neighbors): This system connects adjacent points on the Chinese clock, pairing Hand meridians with their immediately neighboring Foot meridians (e.g., Hand *Tai Yin* Lung balances Foot *Jue Yin* Liver).[1]

These five systems are like five doors that enter the same room from different angles. By learning the key to open each door, the acupuncturist will be able to access any location of the body from any direction. Even if one door is closed, there are other options to open.

---

1. Acupuncture 1,2,3.

Triangulation

Triangulate the chosen points of a treatment in such a way whereby they combine their individual effects to be greater than the sum of their parts. If a treatment is targeting a specific channel, then each point chosen should directly relate to that sick channel. A perfectly triangulated treatment can exert a synergistic effect from multiple directions all at once. They may set out from different locations, but they all reach the same destination and conclusion together. This creates more leverage toward the desired effect, like increasing the arm length of a lever.

For example, if we want to treat the Stomach channel and we only have four needles, we can choose a point from the following four channels:

LI, PC, SP, ST

All four of these channels treat the Stomach channel from four different directions; they represent four different connections to the Foot Yang Ming.

If we want to treat the Bladder channel and we only have four needles, we can choose a point from the following four channels:

SI, LU, KD, BL

All four of these channels treat the Bladder channel from four different directions; four different connections to the Foot Tai Yang.

These systems of channel connectivity originate from the ancient mathematical understanding of the body, forming the six pairs of the twelve Jingmai acupuncture channels. These are purely examples of channels which can be chosen, but the creative potential and individual context means that every treatment offers a unique possibility to find a novel solution within the confines of acupuncture theory and individual point selection.

The Ears

The ear is a prime example of a microcosmic hologram of the entire organism. Various systems have been created for mapping out the relationship between the ear and the human body. One way to approach the ear is to use these systems as a general guide.

However, at some point we must leave the map behind and confront the physical reality in front of us. The most powerful way to approach the ear is through physical inspection. This will tell us valuable information which we can then relate back to what we understand from our guides and our maps.

What do we see when we look at the ear? We should look for areas of abnormality. Dark veins, inflammation, red capillaries, dark splotches, etc. Anything which could represent an irregular or pathological Qi somewhere in the body is possibly reflected and represented in the ear. These are treatment locations. Treat these spots as the bullseye on a target.

Particularly when there is a red capillary or a dark vein, we should allow the removal of stagnant blood when the needle is removed. If blood flows out of the point, this is representative of the restoration of normal Qi and blood dynamics or inflammatory regulation in the area for which that zone mirrors in the body. The ears require extreme precision as they are a small target. They offer us a great opportunity to practice needling without a guide tube, which I find can produce higher accuracy when needling the smallest of vessels.

Liquid Crystals

"Life is water dancing to the tune of solids."
Albert Szent- Györgyi

Since we are water-based bioforms, we inherit the fundamental aspects of water in our biology. The nature of water is to spontaneously create liquid-crystal lattices and pathways, and this enables lower-resistance energy flows to emerge throughout the architecture of our being. When it comes to acupuncture, this liquid-crystalline energy matrix is accessed through the fascial connective tissues, within which acupuncture points reside.

Fascia, which is the liquid-crystalline connective tissue matrix enveloping our entire bodies, is an essential component which makes it possible for the mechanotransductive signals of acupuncture to initiate system-wide modulatory effects. It enables us to experience the De Qi sensation, which is an observable artifact of the activation of this network.

"Liquid crystallinity gives organisms their characteristic flexibility, exquisite sensitivity and responsiveness, thus optimizing the rapid noiseless intercommunication that enables the organism to function as a coherent coordinated whole."
Mae-wan Ho

The acupuncture needle connects with and winds around collagen fibers, causing distortions in the extra-cellular matrix, eliciting physiological responses.[1] The fascia in this way acts as the ground substance of an organism-wide meta-communication system which connects all of the major Psychoneuroendoimmune (PNEI) systems of the body.

The harmonizing effects of acupuncture are like a system-wide spontaneous liquid crystalline metamorphosis which results in more stable, efficient, and functional formations. Acupuncture changes the rhythm and the tune, and the body spontaneously dances into a new configuration.

---

1. Mechanical signaling through connective tissue: a mechanism for the therapeutic effect of acupuncture.

Channels as Zones

Channels are not just linear, two-dimensional lines on a map or poster hanging on a wall. They are multi-dimensional zones of highly complex activity where a tremendous amount of life is occurring at all moments. When we look at a map of geography we don't assume that the lines separating the countries actually exist in the world, and yet sometimes people project that assumption onto the map of the acupuncture channels.

The reality is much more rich and complex. The terrain of the body, being multidimensional, is a multitude of moving energies and substances, all interacting and inexorably interconnected. Membranes pushing and undulating against one another, an infinite dance of molecular complexity pulsating in rhythm with itself, unified by the overarching harmony of the organism as a whole. To engage with a channel is to directly influence and cause a change to the entire fractal web, all of the systems and subsystems, the organs and networks, the electromagnetic substances and energy flows which together comprise the unified physiological system.

It is like an entire physiological river basin, from the mountains to the valley, the main river channel down to all of its minute branching tributaries. The channel is the whole ecosystem of teeming vibrant life which thrives along the life-giving waters. All of the various cells, skin and connective tissues, blood, Qi, and organs form the topography of the channel network, from the surface to the depths. The infinity of the body can be stimulated by a single well-placed needle which activates the Qi of a channel.

Channels each cover vast zones of the body, like fractal planes or faces of a crystalline structure. These 3D zones or domains encompass the surface and the depths of the body, from the skin and hair down through all of the tissues, as well as into and through all of the organ networks.

Each channel represents the fractal geometric relationship which it holds relative to the rest of the body and the physiological areas which they encompass are the most immediately influenced by stimulating them with acupuncture. But they also branch, intersect, connect, and form relationships with one another through mathematical systems such as Yin Yang and Wu Xing, enabling non-local, quasi-quantum effects to take place across the fractal physiological geometry.

Diagnosing the Sick Channel

"Don't just stare at disease. Begin by knowing the evil and the primary Qi and which channels are diseased. For illness, know its origins. First, know which channels are diseased. Then treat them at those origins."
Ling Shu, Chapter 3

Diagnosing the sick channel is the first step for the treatment of pain. "The term 'sick channel' refers to the affected channel. Imbalances can manifest along a sick channel as simply as pain, swelling, or rashes."[1] Symptoms can arise which follow specific patterns according to the channel's internal organ location and function. Signs can show up such as changes in complexion, particular sounds, or particular behaviors. The tongue and the pulse will reflect and resonate. Understanding the various ways to diagnose is important to identify the source and location of the problem.

Without a focused, accurate, rational diagnosis based on the Jing Luo theory of acupuncture channels, then we are just inserting needles at random and hoping for positive results. If we cannot take account of the state of the Qi, then how will we know how to correct the imbalance? Even if we target a muscle or release a trigger point, a deeper issue may still be unresolved; this deeper root causes the propensity for the issue to arise in the first place. This root cause must be sought out and resolved or the propensity will remain and the branch will arise once again.

"Clarify the branch and the root; consider piercing the channels shallowly or deeply. The branch and the root are not limited to a single aspect; there is the branch and root of the six channels, there is the branch and root of Heaven, Earth, Yin and Yang, there is the branch and root of the transmission of disease. Therefore, regarding the human body; then the exterior is the

> *branch, the interior is the root; Yang is the branch, Yin is the root; the Yang bowels are the branch, the Yin viscera are the root; the viscera and bowels located interiorly are the root, the channels and collaterals located exteriorly are the branch."*
> *The Ode of Mysterious Indications, from the Zhenjiu Dacheng*

Without understanding the topography of the body and the pathways of the Jing Mai channels, it is like wandering blindly along the body, or being lost hiking in the mountains or wilderness without a map. If we know the map and how to read it then we can know where we are and we can find the disease's origin. If we can figure that out, then we can deduce the corresponding places that must be treated and which will be the most effective points for eliciting a cure.

---

1. Dr. Tan's Strategy of Twelve Magical Points.

Rivers of Qi

Jīngmài 經脈

"It is simply impossible that there is a place not passed through by the qi. This is like the flow of water, like the movement of sun and moon – they will never stop."
Ling Shu, Chapter 17

What are the acupuncture channels? The conduit vessels which underlie the theory of acupuncture? Through which the Qi is said to 'flow' endlessly?

The body is in a state of perpetual activity on every level. For example, blood flows through the circulatory system, branches off into capillaries, and reaches even the most minute corners of our being where it provides nourishment to cells. In the cellular and extracellular environments there are fluid exchanges and materials being transported across membranes at all times and in all places. The nervous system is continually sending electrical messages throughout every aspect of the organism from the periphery to the central nervous system and back. The activity of Qi continues unabated in all of these multitude of forms, and more. Just like the water of a river, its movement and flow never ceases. The universe is in a constant state of thermodynamic and energetic motion, and this applies to our physiological systems as well.

"Earth has twelve rivers. Man has twelve major channels."
Ling Shu, Chapter 71

On earth, life as we know it, and human civilization, springs up around rivers and river basins. The life giving waters provide the energetic resources for life to occur on its most basic level. In the same way, our water-based bodies follow morphological pathways in their growth and development, akin to physiological rivers. The human body develops according to predetermined mathematical and electromagnetic patterns. The bones, muscles, tendons, arteries, and the rest of the structures of the body follow fractal design principles. We can observe the pathways of their connectivity on a general level by observing the patterns of the development of the human form: such as how the connective tissues and muscles form connective fascial planes, along with all the supportive circulatory and nervous structures following along and innervating the system.

Fractal structures are extremely effective at filling space, and physiological structures do this to maximize efficiency. They form into similar patterns as a river basin does; the main river conduit branches off into multitudes of fractal tributaries, continually becoming ever smaller as the magnification of the landscape increases. We can witness the fractality of the body at every level. The acupuncture channels are the *rivers* of substance, form, and physiological activity and processes. They describe the general interconnectivity which is on display and by whose principles the body forms itself.

> *"From the tips of the hands, Yáng advances and Yīn retreats. From the tips of the feet, Yáng retreats and Yīn advances. Thus uniting the beginning and end of the six channels."*
> *The Lǐ Family of Nánfēng's Supplementation and Drainage, from the Zhenjiu Dacheng*

The characters of Jingmai hold etymological value in that they help to describe the vision which the ancients had about the body. The character *Jing* pictorially represents the longitudinal warp of threads, invoking the symbolism of woven textiles. The character *Mai* pictorially represents the veins and arteries found in flesh or similarly in the arterials of the leaves of plants. Together they form Jingmai, which are the main longitudinal threads, the fleshy warp of the human body through which the arteries and conduits of the organism follow and physiological structures conform.

Jingmai are not just abstract lines on a map, or singular 'tubes' by which Qi flows like water through a hose. They are entire fractalized networks, akin to river basins, by which the entire amalgamated physiological structure forms interconnectedly and intertwined. Qi flows everywhere through this structure; from the skin to the bones, exteriorly and interiorly, in every manner, by means of every microscopic and macroscopic pathway and substance identified and yet to be discovered. It is these networks of physiological substance and activity which acupuncture seeks to ‘tap into’ in order to alter the entire fractal river basin network of the human organism.

Fractal River Basins

River networks are naturally self-organizing fractal formations which optimize the flow of water across landscapes. This fractal structure provides a universal solution to the distribution of resources by filling space efficiently. They organize themselves to minimize dissipation and optimize flow power.

The fractal mathematical laws which govern the way that rivers branch mirror the ratios found in mammalian vascular networks. This fractal complexity provides powerful resilience and bestows anti-fragility to our systems and efficient flow of nourishment and energy to reach throughout our entire three-dimensional being.

> "In reality, a river's basic shape is not a line but a tree. A river is, in essence, a thing that branches... Although it flows inwards towards its trunk, in geological time it grew, and continues to grow, outward, like an organism, from its ocean outlet to its many headwaters. In the vernacular of a new science, it is fractal, its structure echoing itself on all scales, from river to stream to brook to creek to rivulet, branches too small to name and too many to count."[1]

Just as river networks naturally configure themselves into space-filling fractal branches to minimize energy dissipation and stream power, modern research has identified meridians as low hydraulic resistance channels.[2] The fascial connective tissue web is a continuous, volume-filling fractal network that interpenetrates all muscles, organs, and nerves. The flow of Qi and interstitial fluid is the river, the three-dimensional fascial system is the topographical river basin that dictates its path. Acupuncture points lie on different topological parts of the basin: in the mountainous regions, at the emergent springs, along different stages of the river's flow, in the valleys and the hollow basins, or among the seas where all rivers eventually travel to.

Pathology in the river basin is like the emergence of stagnation, blockage, or obstruction somewhere in the natural flow. By using acupuncture to send a fractal wave through the river basin, we can potentially clear obstructions and reopen the parts of the network which were at risk of losing their fractal complexity.

---

1. Nature's Chaos.
2. Meridian Studies in China: A Systematic Review.

Tributaries

Luòmài 絡脈

Where the Jingmai are the main longitudinal channels of the physiological river network, the Luomai are the crisscrossing latitudinal, tertiary network vessels which interlace and interweave with the main waters of the body.

The Chinese character *Luo* is composed of the silk radical on the left and a phonetic element on the right. Etymologically, it translates to unreeled silk, hemp, cotton fiber, a net, or to attach, evoking the image of a fibrous mesh, the stringy pith of citrus fruits, or the interlacing threads of a loofah sponge.

Functionally, the Luomai act as reservoirs and overflow ditches for the main physiological rivers. When the main channels are overwhelmed with excess Qi, blood, or pathogenic evils, the overflow spills into the Luomai. This fractal-like structure helps to absorb shocks to the system and distribute the load. Because the *luo* collaterals are where external pathogens (like wind, cold, or physical trauma) easily become trapped, they frequently suffer from blood stasis and coagulation. And because the *Luomai* are located superficially in the body, they are visible to the naked eye and serve as a direct diagnostic window into the body's internal state.

> *"The conduit vessels are usually invisible... All the vessels that can be seen are network vessels."*
> *Ling Shu, Chapter 10*

The general rule of classical practice is that network vessels must always be pierced where knots have formed and where there is very much dark, engorged blood. This instantly relieves localized pressure, releases the trapped pathogenic evil, and restores the free flow of Qi within the main river system.

Luo points form the basis of the classical "Host and Guest" point combination. In this strategy, the Yuan-source point of the primarily affected channel (the Host) is combined with the Luo-collateral point of its coupled channel (the Guest). Functionally, this strategy perfectly aligns with the architecture of the channel system. While the Yuan-source point stabilizes the main subterranean 'river' (the primary channel), the Luo-collateral point regulates the superficial 'tributaries' (i.e., the collateral vessels).

Transports

Shū 輸

The Chinese character Shū translates roughly as 'transport', or the process of carrying or hauling something off. These points access the Qi of the channel vessels or the organ hubs and modulate excesses or deficiencies. Distal Shu points treat the conduit vessels while back Shu points reach the Qi of the Zang (depot) and Fu (palace) organs which lie proximal to them.

On a general level, transport points are somewhat synonymous with acupuncture points in general: all acupuncture points essentially function as a form of Qi transport. But on a more specific level, transport points as a group are classified as their own subset due to their recognized uses for treating a myriad of ailments. Because of their potency, needling the distal or the back Shu points is the first of the nine methods of needling spoken of in the *Ling Shu*.[1]

> *"The human body has transporter holes like a room has doors."*
> *Yao Shaoyu, Su Wen Commentary, Chapter 42*

By opening these doors and valves, the transport acupuncture points modulate the flow of Qi throughout the body, through the channels and organ systems, similar to how water flow is regulated through dykes, levees, or dams.

---

1. Ling Shu, Chapter 7.

Distal Transports

"The names well, brook, stream, channel, and confluence reflect the nature of the flow of Qi at each of these points. The ancient Chinese likened the flow of Qi in the channels to the flow of water from its source in the mountains to its home in the sea."
A Practical Dictionary of Chinese Medicine

The theory of the Five Shu-Points (transporting points) is a profound example of classical Chinese medicine projecting the macrocosmic environmental world onto the human microcosm. Ancient Chinese naturalists mapped the geography of the earth directly onto human anatomy, viewing the body's channels as subterranean rivers and waterways that transport vital Qi and blood, much like the great rivers of China irrigate the land. The theory of the distal shu points really came into its own with the influence of *Nan Jing*.

"That which emerges is the well, the well resembles a spring of water. That which glides is the spring, the spring resembles a pool of water. That which pours is the stream, the stream resembles a transport corridor of water. That which circulates is the river, the river resembles the flow of water. That which enters is the sea, the sea resembles the returning of water. All take their meaning from water."
The Song of the Wells, Springs, Streams, Sources, Rivers, and Seas, from the Zhenjiu Dacheng

The five categories of points each capture a specific morphological stage of this physiological river, dictating their clinical usage.[1]

1. Jing-Well Points
   - Nature: The point at which the Qi emanates is known as the jing-well. The Qi here is compared to water bubbling up from a well. Because the physical flesh is thin here, the Qi is shallow and narrow, yet it is extremely volatile, dynamic, and rapidly changing.

   - Practical Application: In classical symptomatology, they treat "fullness below the Heart" (Liver pathogen). Due to the highly dynamic and volatile nature of the Qi at the extremities, these points are the most powerful on the body for restoring consciousness, rescuing collapse, and clearing intense heat. Furthermore, because they are at the absolute extremities, they are uniquely effective at treating the uppermost, opposite ends of the channels.

2. Ying-Spring Points
   - Nature: "The point at which the Qi glides is known as the ying-spring". The Qi here dashes forward, streaming like a small brook or the rising water of a spring. They are the second or penultimate points on the extremities.

   - Practical Application: Classically, they are indicated for "heat in the body" (Heart pathogen) and changes in the complexion. In practice, Ying-Spring points are primarily used to clear pathogenic heat and fire from their respective channels and organs. This is because, according to Five Phase theory, the Ying-Spring points on Yin channels belong to Fire, and on Yang channels they belong to Water, giving them an unmatched ability to subdue heat. Unlike Jing-Well points, their therapeutic reach covers diseases along the entire course of the channel, not just the uppermost tips.

3. Shu-Stream Points
   - Nature: "The point at which the Qi pours through is known as the shu-stream". At this stage, the water deepens and pours downward, resembling a stream growing wide enough to transport vessels and accumulate energy.

   - Practical Application: They are classically indicated for "heaviness of the body and pain of the joints" (Spleen pathogen), making them the primary points for treating dampness and painful obstruction (Bi syndrome) anywhere in the body. Crucially, on all the Yin channels, the Shu-Stream points are functionally identical to the Yuan-Source points. Therefore, they are considered the single most important points on the Yin channels for supplementing and harmonizing their respective solid Zang organs.

4. Jing-River Points
    - Nature: "The point at which the Qi flows is known as the jing-river". The Qi here moves uninterrupted, resembling a deep, wide river that has generated a huge track. They are generally located at or proximal to the wrist and ankle joints.
    - Practical Application: The classics prescribe these points for cough, dyspnea, chills, and fever (Lung pathogen), as well as diseases manifesting as changes in the patient's voice. Additionally, they have a powerful action in treating diseases of the sinews and bones, such as contracted sinews or bone painful obstruction.

5. He-Sea Points
    - Nature: "The point at which the Qi enters inwards is known as the he-sea". Situated close to the large joints of the elbows and knees, the Qi here runs extremely deep and broad, acting like an estuary flowing into the sea. It is the place where the superficial channel Qi plunges deep into the body to unite with the internal organs.
    - Practical Application: They are classically indicated for counterflow Qi and diarrhea (Kidney pathogen) and diseases of the Stomach resulting from irregular eating and drinking. In practice, they are the most important points for treating the internal Fu bowels, particularly the intestines, digestion, and urinary system. Furthermore, the He-Sea points on the Yang channels are heavily utilized to treat diseases of the skin.

---

1. Nan Jing, Chapter 68

Back Transports

"The shu points are situated in the yang region [the back], they may be used to treat yin diseases"
Nan Jing, Chapter 67

The Back Shu points have been utilized extensively since ancient times. These points are discussed at length throughout the *Su Wen* and the *Ling Shu*. Needling the Shu points is known as 'Transport Needling' and it is the first of the 'Nine Needling Methods' mentioned in the *Ling Shu*. They are extremely important points to study, master and utilize in practice because they have a broad application.

"The transporter holes of the depots, five on both sides, these ten holes are employed to drain the heat of the five depots."
Wang Bing, Su Wen Commentary Chapter 32

As stated in the classics, the Back Shu points clear heat and inflammation. This is true because of their location at the surface, making them easy candidates for the use of venting techniques for the exterior, yang section of the body. Their functional locations serve multiple uses, however, and the classics also recommend them for treating the Yin organ systems — the Zang organs.

"For treating the depots, treat their transporters."
Su Wen Chapter 38

These points anatomically lie directly above their respective organs, making them useful for clearing deeper levels of heat, inflammation, and Xie Qi, beyond just the exterior. This can sometimes even be seen visually where a patient has observable redness and erythema over the needled back Shu points. Allow this heat to vent out and dissipate during the treatment.

> *One pierces those transporters located near the [affected] depot because it is there that the depot Qi accumulates. It is there that the Qi of the depots meets and effuses."*
> *Wu Kun and Wang Bing, Su Wen Commentaries, Chapter 55*

Furthermore, these points have the capacity to clear excesses from the channel vessel networks, enabling them to engage with the basins of Qi and Blood in the body. These are powerful points to have in our repertoire and there are daily opportunities to use them in the clinic.

> *"When the vessels are full and big, quickly pierce the transporters on the back."*
> *Su Wen, Chapter 36*

Aggressive Energy

One of the greatest acupuncture treatment protocols comes from the *Ling Shu* where needling the Back Shu points is commonly cited for a variety of conditions. This treatment strategy later became a cornerstone of J.R. Worsley's 'Five Element Acupuncture' system. He describes 'aggressive energy' as Qi "which has become contaminated or polluted." This is essentially synonymous with the classical idea of Xie Qi.

> *"Aggressive energy can also be described as evil or unhealthy (xie) Qi, as opposed to upright or healthy (zheng) Qi."*
> *J.R. Worsley*

Broadly clearing Xie Qi from the channels and Zang Fu organs is possible using this treatment strategy. The virtues of the Back Shu points is that they deeply interconnect with the organ systems of the body. By needling each of the Zang Back Shu points, Xie Qi is vented from the system. For this, shallow needling is done in order to facilitate the venting of Xie Qi through these transportation holes.

This is a wonderful treatment to begin a longer course of acupuncture with. By clearing lingering Xie Qi first, it creates a strong foundation for future acupuncture treatments to be even more successful.

> *"One must first drain, then supplement. This is called 'first draining evil Qi, then supplementing true Qi'. This is the secret formula not passed on by the earlier masters."*
> *Supplementation and Drainage from the Classic of Spiritual Correspondence, from the Zhenjiu Dacheng*

A confirmation that Xie Qi was present and is being actively vented is the formation of erythema around the Back Shu points that are needled. It is ideal to retain the needles until all of the inflammatory Xie Qi has been removed. As confirmed by the classics, this is a profound treatment which should not be underestimated!

Confluences

Huì 會

Due to the crisscrossing nature of the Jingmai and Luomai acupuncture channels, network vessels, and fascia, we can be on the lookout for important confluence points. These are areas of physiological importance and powerful sites of acupuncture therapy.

Hui translates as a meeting, gathering, union, or an association. These are the areas where Qi flows meet, combine, and intersect. Acupuncture points in these locations can access the Qi and *waters* of multiple fractal physiological river basins at once from a single location. They are like the geographical points where two or more rivers unite.

> *"These eight acupoints penetrate to the origin and end of the eight vessels, linking up to the eight confluences, and are inherently the guiding principle of a human. Like a fishing net has a main rope."*
> *The Ode of Mysterious Indications, from the Zhenjiu Dacheng*

Because of these natural junctions, confluence points have access points to large flows of Qi. They are vortexes of physiological potential which can be utilized to influence multiple large swathes of physiological terrain simultaneously. The *Su Wen* specifically recommend these points for treating the Fu organs:

> *"For treating the palaces, treat their [respective] confluences."*
> *Su Wen Chapter 38*

Oceans and Seas

Hǎi 海

"Man has four seas and twelve river-like channels. All rivers flow to the sea."
Ling Shu, Chapter 33

Just as "all roads lead to Rome", the channels of the body flow all throughout the surface as well as the depths of the body where they form vast networks of tendon, bone, flesh, fascia, blood, and bodily fluids. These networks enmesh the central physiological 'metropolitan' hubs or thoroughfares of the bodily empire. Oceans and seas are vast bodies of water. Metaphorically, these vast oceans and seas of Qi represent rich local sources and reservoirs of the organism's vitality, energy, substance, function and potential.

"People have four seas... the Sea of Marrow, the Sea of Blood, the Sea of Qi, and the Sea of Water and Grains."
Ling Shu, Chapter 33

Each sea thus governs large portions of physiological activity according to their associations. The *Ling Shu* identifies four seas and offers us powerful points through which we might access them and regulate the physiological correlates which they represent:

The Stomach; the Sea of Water and Grains - ST 30 & ST 36

The Brain; the Sea of Marrow - GV 16 & GV 20

The Chest center; the Sea of Qi - CV 17, ST 9, GV 14 & GV 15

The Chong Mai; the Sea of Blood - BL 10, ST37 & ST 39

River Conditions

Have you ever walked along a river and saw a downed tree, creating a blockage along the river pathway? The debris impedes the normal flow of the river, creating areas where stagnant, sludgy water pools form, collect and grow. This is a metaphor for what happens physiologically when the normal healthy flow is disrupted in our tissues, channels, and channel vessels.

> *"When heaven and earth are warm and harmonious, then the main waters are quiet and calm. When heaven is cold and the earth is frozen, then the main waters congeal so that their flow is impeded. When heaven has summerheat and the earth is hot, then the main waters gush forth as if boiling and overflow. When a sudden wind rises violently, then the main waters gush up like breakers and rise like ridges in the fields."*
> *Su Wen, Chapter 27*

Just as the harmonious flow of water is disrupted by these different conditions, so is the body, which is composed primarily of water. The presence of various pathogens or influences can disrupt the normal structure, function, and state of the channel vessels and pathways. This can cause structural and functional degradation and the development of disharmonies, resulting in various symptoms such as pain. Think of how powerfully our bodies react when we are exposed to extreme heat, cold, wind conditions, dampness, or dryness. Imagine how water reacts when exposed to these influences in nature. Inevitably, these conditions will affect the 'waters' of the human body and result in adverse diseased 'river conditions' throughout the conduits and vessels.

> *"The six conduits are streams; the intestines and stomach are the sea. The nine orifices are where Qi flows like water."*
> *Su Wen, Chapter 5*

Our bodies can develop conglomerations or accumulations and masses. Tissues can become taut and unable to release or so slack that they can no longer contract. Blood can coagulate, harden, and stagnate. All cells of our body rely not just on blood flow but also on mucous membranes and fluid extracellular environments. If there is water retention, blood stagnation, inflammation, external pathogens, or phlegmy stagnant accumulations, physiological function will inevitably be injured. The opposite is also true — if there is deficiency or a lack of blood, Qi, or fluids, the banks of the rivers will run dry and erosion will commence.

Obstructions

Bì 痺

"The skillful acupuncturist can take hold of the disease in the same way one pulls out thorns, washes out stains, unties knots, or breaches obstructions. Disease, although chronic, still can be ended. Those who say diseases are incurable have not mastered the technique of acupuncture."
Ling Shu, Chapter 1

Part of the purpose of acupuncture is to remove obstructions, expel pathogenic influences, and reestablish dynamic and harmonious flow in areas where blockages have emerged. This reestablishes the body's upright Qi and proper functioning. The concept of *Bi*, translated as "block," "obstruction," or "impediment," is a central concept for a slew of pathologies. It describes a group of diseases caused by the invasion and stagnation of exogenous environmental pathogens in the body's superficial layers and meridian network, which, if unresolved, can penetrate deeply into the internal organs.

"The three Qi of wind, cold, and damp all arrive in miscellaneous ways and combine to produce Bi. When wind Qi prevails, this is migratory Bi. When cold Qi prevails, this is painful Bi. And when damp Qi prevails, this is fixed Bi."
Su Wen, Chapter 43

As noted in the *Ling Shu*, the "Yangming channel is abundant in Qi and blood". This natural energetic abundance makes Yangming points ideal for promoting the circulation needed to resolve numbness, paralysis, stiffness, and pain in the limbs. A definitive classical pairing is provided in the *Secrets of the Heavenly Star*, which explicitly asks and answers: "Cold wind damp painful obstruction, where do you needle? First choose Huantiao GB30, then Yanglingquan GB34".

ST31 is a pivotal point (functionally equivalent to LI15 on the arm) used to regulate the circulation of qi and blood for the entire leg, making it essential for cold painful obstruction of the knees and atrophy. KD3 is specifically noted for treating heel pain caused by painful obstruction. The extra points Baxie are highly effective for clearing heat, stiffness, swelling, and painful obstruction in the fingers.

The Dao Ma needling technique as a targeted grouping significantly improves the effectiveness of treating Bi syndromes. The primary way the Dao Ma technique enhances treatment potency is by leveraging the holographic "Taiji" correspondence (the concept that a small part of the body mirrors the whole). Dao Ma groups are frequently combined with kinetic movement of the painful location. The concentrated, high-potency stimulation generated by the Dao Ma cluster forcefully breaks the local stagnation in the sick meridian as the patient moves, often resulting in immediate relief.

A common clinical error when treating complex Bi syndromes is applying too many scattered needles across the body to chase multiple symptoms, which can confuse the treatment signal and overcomplicate the point selection. The Dao Ma technique solves this by consolidating the treatment into a highly potent, localized cluster.

Clearing

Tōng 通

Some of the meanings of the Chinese character *tōng* include "to go through to, to penetrate, to clear, to open; to communicate; to free or unblock." If acupuncture is an act of governing the bodily empire and the system back to a state of functional order, *tōng* names the condition being restored — the unimpeded, continuous flow of Qi, blood, fluids, and bodily resources, enabling communication through every level of the system.

> *"It is said of the needle's stem, though minute as a hair, it can penetratingly clear all of the channel's Qì and blood, balance heat and cold of the five viscera, and can regulate excesses and deficiencies of the six bowels."*
> *The Ode of Mysterious Indications, from the Zhenjiu Dacheng*

In terms of the acupuncture channels, *tōng* holds the sense of clearing or opening them. When the channels become obstructed, rough, and blocked, this results in many forms of disease emerging. In our youth, the channels are all clear and free-flowing — this is the optimal state of channel health. Obstructions of all kinds develop due to one's diet, external factors such as cold or heat, poor habits, traumatic injuries, or just naturally with age. Because of this, clearing, connecting, or opening the channels is an essential aspect of acupuncture treatment. When communication is reestablished, the natural healing, rejuvenating mechanisms of the body can resume.

> *"...One must certainly connect the Qì and clear the channels, and furthermore, use the methods of opposing and complying to enable the Qì and blood to pass through clearly and the channels and collaterals to reconnect and replenish."*
> *The Ode of Mysterious Indications, from the Zhenjiu Dacheng*

The cosmos itself is a dynamic continuum of the interpenetrating alternations of Yin and Yang. When this process unfolds unimpeded, this is, in essence, *tong.* As this process reveals itself in manifold ways physiologically in the body, such as through the endless circulation of Qi and blood, it is also an important term for health, medicine, and acupuncture. One of the main tasks of the acupuncturist is to locate where circulation and communication have become blocked and congealed, and to open, regulate, and clear it using acupuncture's methods.

> *"To open [the flow of] the Qi, and to regulate it, this is the Way of this."*
> *Su Wen, Chapter 74*

This concept also speaks to the importance of practices such as Qigong and Daoyin exercises; methods used to nourish one's life. One of the main reasons they are effective is because they open the channels, circulate the Qi, and keep the body free of obstructions and stagnation.

Bodily Ecology

The inner world of the body mirrors the cosmos — it is a microcosm teeming with habitats, its inner ecology as vast and varied as Earth's own terrains. This paradigm permeates the names of the acupuncture points themselves. And this sort of fractal holographic vision of the world is echoed in the language of the classics, where they map the body according to natural formations.

> *"Where the large conduits meet, these locations are called 'large valleys'. The 'twelve divisions' are the twelve conduit-vessel sections. Where the small network vessels meet, these locations are called 'small ravines'."*
> *Wang Bing, Su Wen Chapter 10 Commentary*

Like charting a landscape, diagnostics such as pulse and tongue examination reveal the body's terrain and the state of the Qi to the practitioner. What is the state of their physiological ecosystem? An ecosystem which is in disorder experiences harsh conditions, a loss of diversity, and ultimately ecological collapse. An ecosystem in harmony is vibrant, lush, and rich with life. Its waters flow clear and pure, nourishing every corner of the land with Qi at the appropriate times. On a microscopic level, the flow of Qi should penetrate to every corner of our extracellular matrix, nourishing the individual cells themselves.[1]

What are the ecological conditions of our patient? Are they exhibiting the signs of a damp marsh or arid desert conditions? Does dampness mire them with loose stool and edema, signaling Spleen's swamp? Or does dryness parch with brittle hair and cracked skin, hinting at Lung's desert? Cold can grip with the tight, slow pulse of a tundra's chill or heat can flare red on the tongue and face, with a bounding, racing pulse that signals blazing internal fire.

Rivers can constrict to the point where they do not reach their destinations or become stagnant, blocked and obstructed. Does their blood flow struggle to reach their extremities or do we find they have pain and obstruction syndromes in their joints? We can see the parallels between our diagnostic investigations and the inner bodily ecologies.

Marshes, Mountains, Rivers, Valleys, Ravines, Plains, Deserts, Oceans: this is the sort of terrain and language which can be analogous to the ecosystems of our bodies. Not every habitat is suitable for the flourishing of life. As acupuncturists, we must identify the patient's bodily ecology and intervene in order to terraform towards a harmonious state which engenders health and life.

---

1. Is There Volume Transmission Along Extracellular Fluid Pathways Corresponding to the Acupuncture Channels?

Terraforming Environments

Environments change as a rule, and this can occur at varying speeds depending upon the conditions and the variables. Generally speaking, in scenarios where health prevails, a dynamic steady state equilibrium is found and maintained. This is conducive to thermodynamic efficiency and optimal function.

Where the body is viewed as a landscape of rivers, valleys, and varying climates, disease is akin to an ecological crisis. In acute dysfunction, intense fluctuations of volatility and disruption of this harmony result in rapid manifestations of symptoms, as the system attempts to stabilize. In chronic dysfunction, change happens much more slowly over time and it is sometimes less perceptible. That is, until the energetic burden becomes such that the system itself is forced to accommodate and adapt to the stress, unleashing a cascading avalanche of ever worsening chronic symptoms. We can see this fragility occur in external habitats and environments, but we don't always consider its occurrence within the body.

> *"In ancient times, those who knew the way patterned themselves on yin and yang, harmonized with the arts of calculation, ate and drank with moderation, regulated their daily living, and did not overexert themselves, thus they were able to keep body and spirit in harmony and live out their full natural space of life, reaching a hundred years before departing."*
> *Su Wen, Chapter 1*

One of the goals of medicine is to change the environment of the organism to a more ordered, harmonious system or state, which is synonymous with health. This means regulation of the factors which shape the environment within: our habits, our diets, our emotions.

The foods and drinks we consume provide the basic raw materials of our physiology. Our habits and practices accumulate over time like sediments. Powerful emotions carve lines into our faces, reflecting their energetics within through external spontaneous reflexes. Stress and inflammation slowly take their toll on our systems, reflective of the attempt to restore harmony.

The classics also describe various external pathogenic agents which can alter the internal environment and cause disease. For example, harsh and prolonged exposure to the raw elements of wind, cold, and heat can exert a detrimental effect, as our system must expend intense resources to maintain equilibrium. People who are in contact with the extreme elements of nature, such as cold, wind, dampness, dryness or heat, are at a heightened risk of ecological disruption.

Internally, what was once a normal valley can become flooded marshlands, manifesting as edema, loose stool, and damp overgrowths harboring micro-organisms. What was once a fertile field can become a withered desert landscape, manifesting as dry skin, withering hair, and chronic constipation. When harmony of Yin and Yang is lost, our inner landscapes and ecosystems start to break down.

The job of the practitioner is to identify where and what imbalance has occurred and to rectify it. Acupuncture and herbal medicine are powerful tools for terraforming an inner environment which has lost its harmony. Acupuncture handles the riverways and the transportation channels, while herbal medicine fundamentally transforms and terraforms the landscape. By clearing and regulating the channels, the ecosystem can naturally rebalance and harmonize by more effectively transporting resources and expelling waste. By delivering medicinals with their different flavors, natures, and actions, the body acquires the necessary and specific energetic materials it needs to rebuild and to terraform the inner landscape.

The Gates

One of my favorite thought practices is to reverse-engineer acupuncture point protocols. We can consider the point selections and try to dissect the theory and the rationale behind why these points were used. Doing this helps us to understand both the protocol and the individual points better. A common and very potent acupoint formula is the combination of LI4 and LV3, often referred to as the 'four gates'.

For cold, heat, impediment, and pain, simply open the four gates.
The Ode of Mysterious Indications, From the Zhenjiu Dacheng

LI4 is the source point of the large intestine channel. Its classical name is 'Uniting Valley', alluding to both its junction-like location on the hand as well as its energetic interconnectedness. LI4 powerfully activates the upright Qi and circulates it throughout the body. The hand Yangming LI channel has intimate connections to the LU, ST, LV, and KD. The LI channel itself travels to the face and head, and the Yangming converges to traverse large portions of the shoulders, neck, and the entire frontal plane of the face. This gives LI4 broad capabilities to the upper portions of the body. The Yangming is described as having very large quantities of Qi and blood. Personally, I always needle this point using the Master Tung Dao Ma of Linggu and Dabai for maximum effect, unless a patient is extremely weak or sensitive or the Qi is obtained extremely quickly and powerfully with a single needle.

LV3 is also the source point of the Liver channel. Its classical name is 'Extreme Surge' or 'Greatest Thoroughfare'. These source points, by together activating the upright Qi, have powerful regulatory effects on the entire system. The LV channel's connections are to the PC, LI, GB, SI, and LU. The LV channel travels through the lower body, the groin and inguinal region, and into the abdomen, ribs, and hypochondrium, giving it broad capabilities to the lower jiao, organs, and the portions of the bodily terrain traversed by the Liver and Gallbladder. The Jueyin is described as having large quantities of blood, but as Zhu Dan-xi explains, "the Liver governs spreading and draining." Much like LI4, this point can be needled as a Dao Ma with LV2, but I typically only utilize this when a patient displays overt signs of excessive heat.

> *'Four Gates' refers to the six viscera having twelve sources, arising from the four gates, namely, 'Greatest Thoroughfare' LV3 and 'Uniting Valley' LI4.*
> *The Ode of Mysterious Indications, From the Zhenjiu Dacheng*

Holographically speaking, these points are mirror images of one another, existing in anatomically correlated positions on the hand and foot respectively. Taken in sum, these two points alone directly influence eight of the twelve (¾ in total) of the channels through the channel relationships. Their regulatory effects therefore influence most of the organ systems and their respective channel terrain on the upper and lower body, meaning they have far-reaching, broad spectrum actions as points.

They initiate an intense surge of Qi through the body, regulating Jingluo conditions and removing obstructions, hinted to by the name of LV3. It is like opening a pressure valve to release steam, or opening the gates of a dam to release water. They can 'wash away' obstructions in the Jingluo by powerfully circulating upright Qi. By virtue of the LI and LV sharing one another as direct connections channels, their mutual effect is resonant and amplified. Of the Four Gates, *The Manual of Acupuncture* explains: "they are able to vigorously activate the qi and blood and ensure their free and smooth passage throughout the body".

These two points, when needled bilaterally, are commonly called the 'Four Gates'. However, I have found that they are also effective when used as a two-point combination, needled contralaterally from one another, so I just like to call them 'The Gates'. This allows for the acupuncturist to combine another two-point contralateral combination to make a more dynamic and targeted four-point combination.

For example, consider a scenario where a patient has back pain on the Bladder channel. Instead of using the Four Gates, one could create a point combination to target the Taiyang along with reaping the benefit of the Gates, such as:

SI3, LI4

LV3, Bl40

This same concept can be adapted and applied to other situations. If the pain presents on the Gallbladder, one can use points which target the Shaoyang instead, such as:

SJ3, LI4

LV3, GB41

Another way that I like to play with this concept of The Gates is to just treat Yangming and Jueyin together as a whole. This changes the gates from contralateral to bilateral and makes one of the most potent acupuncture points, ST36, interchangeable with LV3 when appropriate. In this combination, LV3 forms a channel relationship with both PC6 and LI4. Likewise, ST has channel connections to both LI and PC points.

LI4, PC6

LV3, ST36

The first two examples are great protocols for back pain or sciatica. The third example is wonderful for regulating emotions, digestion, and the abdominal center. These are just three ideas on how one can flexibly utilize The Gates to create dynamic four-point combinations that go far beyond the static Four Gates. In fact, the possibilities are practically endless for this approach and it can be modified in almost any direction we need. I find that this is one of the most effective targeted approaches to almost any pain condition. I also find it useful for any situation where one seeks to employ strong Qi circulation and channel clearing. They can be paired with other points for a combined treatment strategy or points which bring the treatment actions to other target locations.

Interconnected Systems

Chinese medicine developed one of the first conceptions of the body utilizing a systems theory. The concept of *Zang Fu*, the viscera and the bowels, conceptualizes the organs as dynamic, interrelated functional systems. The organs are not merely biological processors. They are administrative officials in the body's imperial court, each holding a specific office essential to the organism's survival. Understanding the body as interconnected systems helps us engage with the sheer complexity of human physiology in a way which does not fall prey to pure reductionism.

Another way to view the body as interconnected systems is the modern field of psychoneuroendoimmunology (PNEI). PNEI is the study of interactions among the psychological, neurological, endocrine, and immune systems, such as the bidirectional crosstalk and feedback loops which exist between them. What is authentically useful is that these two systems, developed thousands of years apart from entirely different assumptions, arrive at strikingly similar conclusions about the interconnectedness of how the body organizes itself. When held up against each other and used comparatively, both sets of ideas come into sharper focus due to the additional perspectives.

Acupuncture modulates these PNEI systems and initiates physiological cascades which ripple through the whole. This is why it is so effective at influencing complex chronic multi-system disorders, or chronic inflammatory conditions. When a disorder affects multiple systems, a treatment which modulates all of them at once can restore homeostatic flexibility and dynamism. With a single needle, acupuncture's mechanical signal elicits a fascial wave, triggering a hypothalamic-pituitary cascade that shifts the body towards parasympathetic dominance, endocrine and inflammatory modulation, stress reduction, and default mode network deactivation *simultaneously*.

A treatment which targets only one system (like a standard anti-inflammatory drug or a selective serotonin reuptake inhibitor) may temporarily reduce peripheral cytokines or alter local neurotransmitters. However, if the central limbic system remains in a hyper-aroused state, or if peripheral inflammatory responses remain active, the bidirectional nature of the PNEI means the untreated nodes will simply re-initiate the inflammatory cascade and could override the localized treatment.

Acupuncture overcomes this by functioning as a global neuromodulator that simultaneously addresses the central, autonomic, and peripheral components of the feedback loop, effectively issuing a synchronized "reset" command across the entire organism (or, the entire empire). This is a modern way of saying that acupuncture treats the root.

Phlegm

Tán 痰

Phlegm is an interesting topic because it is generated as a result of other pathological processes, but it is also pathological in itself and can create second-order issues. Its nature is that it is sticky, dense, hard to clear, and difficult to penetrate. As stated in the *Manual of Acupuncture*, "chronic disease often involves phlegm."

> *"When the Qi of wind, cold, and dampness have intruded upon the partings of the flesh, (fluid and humor) are oppressed and condensed into foam. When this foam contacts cold, it gathers and, while gathering, it presses and separates the partings of the flesh. This separation produces pain."*
> *Ling Shu, Chapter 27*

The *Ling Shu* description of the formation of foam provides a vivid image of how phlegm is generated. It is the body's own fluids congealing pathologically, causing blockages, obstructions, accumulations, and occluding the channels and collaterals. We can see this happen in the natural world when we walk along a river and observe its flow. We can surely find foamy, congealed areas where obstructions are present, or where a sharp turn causes a pathological buildup of exudate. These areas are clearly differentiated from the parts of the river which flows smoothly. This hints at the true cause of phlegm, and also how to resolve it.

> *"The primary strategy for treating phlegm is to smooth the flow of Qi and keep the passageways of Qi, blood, and body fluids open."*
> *Formulas and Strategies*

Phlegm also results from the congregation of pathogens. "The ability to form biofilms is a universal attribute of bacteria. Biofilms are multicellular communities held together by a self-produced extracellular matrix."[1] These biofilms are intricate microbial communities which form colonies and take residence within our bodies.[2] By developing their own extracellular matrix of phlegmy biofilm, they are better able to evade the host's immune response, as well as insulate themselves from antimicrobials. For this reason, phlegm is often present and relevant to consider whenever one is dealing with lingering, chronic, and hard to treat issues. This is where phlegm interfaces with Gu Syndrome and hard to treat, lingering pathogens.[3]

---

1. Biofilms.
2. Understanding Biofilms.
3. Covid: A Modern Form of Gu Syndrome

Entropy

Entropy is the statistical measure of disorder, unpredictability, and irreversibility within a system. Applied to living organisms, it is the thermodynamic framing for understanding how acupuncture supports health by modulating entropy gradients. When entropy rises, it represents a state of chaos and disorder in the system. When entropy becomes too low, it manifests as rigidity and the inability for the organism to adapt or change. Ultimately, from a thermodynamic perspective, death represents the final situation where entropy crosses an irreversible threshold in either direction — rising past the organism's capacity to counteract chaotic dissipation, or falling so low that the system loses the flexibility needed to adapt and change.

> *"A living organism can only hold off the state of maximum entropy, that being death, by absorbing negative entropy, or negentropy, from the environment."*
> *Erwin Schrödinger*

Living organisms are open systems, which means they exchange matter and energy with their environment. This lets them locally reduce internal entropy generated from normal metabolic processes by continuously exporting it outward. In a healthy state, inflammation is a highly coordinated, temporary mechanism used to restore homeostasis. When an open system is deprived of energy and becomes vacuous internally, it becomes less capable of managing internal disorder. This can manifest as uncontrolled, chronic inflammation, which serves as a central mechanism driving the degradation of health and the onset of disease. A system in this state also becomes extremely vulnerable to external invading pathogens; its boundaries and constraints become porous and weakened, its defenses chaotic and in disarray, less capable of fending off Xie Qi.

"Vacuity evils simply mean pathological vacuity or the evil of vacuity. Thieving evils have no way to enter [the body] unless vacuity evils have [already] struck."
Li Dong-Yuan, Pi Wei Lun

A healthy biological system relies on fractal-like variability to adapt. Health exists in a state of criticality or edge-of-chaos dynamics — balanced entropy with rich, fractal/multifractal variability, metastable states, and efficient information processing. These properties allow self-organization, adaptability, and homeostasis without collapsing into pathological levels of order or chaos.

Disease is in many ways a loss of physiological complexity. Illness can be viewed, in thermodynamic terms, as a (usually reversible) tipping or strain of the entropy balance. In diseased states our systems become either rigidly periodic (pathologically regular) or completely uncorrelated (like white noise); both conditions represent an entropic failure. Chronic high entropy yields chaotic, inflammatory, uncorrelated noise, a loss of boundaries, and vulnerability. Pathological low entropy manifests as overly rigid, periodic, stereotyped patterns with an accompanying loss of variability. Examples include locked-in repetitive firing, fibrosis, or rigid autonomic balance. Both of these scenarios reduce physiological complexity.

When available free energy declines, the system experiences a drop in its action efficiency, meaning it can no longer execute internal processes such as metabolic reactions effectively. The organism becomes increasingly fragile, structurally compromised, and less adaptable to external environmental fluctuations. If the imbalance remains within the system's resilience, feedback loops and repair processes re-establish control and the entropy falls back toward the healthy range. If the imbalance becomes self-reinforcing and crosses irreversible thresholds, the trajectory continues and the flow of Qi ceases completely, the system becomes entirely vacuous internally or inflamed to an unsustainable level, and the process of spontaneous self-organization grinds to a halt; ultimately these situations result in death.

"Entropy is the price of structure."
Ilya Prigogine

Acupuncture treatment restores optimal complexity and critical dynamics, evidenced in neuroimaging by enhanced interregional functional connectivity (especially in the default mode and sensorimotor networks) and restored sympathetic/parasympathetic balance.[1] Acupuncture can be understood as injecting negentropy (information) into a biological system; it is a low-energy, high-information input. A high-energy system can be reorganized by a low-energy message carrying very high information.

> *"The essential thing in metabolism is that the organism succeed in freeing itself from all the entropy it cannot help producing while alive, much like the wake left by a passing ship."*
> *Erwin Schrödinger*

By actively restoring the body to a state of optimal criticality and recovering the multifractal properties of the system, acupuncture restores the flexible, self-organized order of the interconnected physiological networks that allows the organism to remain adaptable, action-efficient, and homeodynamic, far from thermodynamic equilibrium. So I would say that acupuncture is fundamentally a technique to modulate entropy, guiding biological systems back to critical states of healthy complexity.

---

1. Decoding the mechanisms of acupuncture by neuroimaging: an integrated review from networks to molecules.

Inflammation

"It is by avoiding the rapid decay into the inert state of 'equilibrium' that an organism appears so enigmatic... How does the living organism avoid decay?"
Erwin Schrödinger

Erwin Schrödinger famously stated that a living organism can only maintain its highly organized state and ward off death by continuously drawing negative entropy (negentropy) from its environment. Living systems are open, out-of-equilibrium thermodynamic entities. They preserve their highly intricate structural order by locally reducing their internal entropy. This process requires a massive, ongoing expenditure of metabolic energy (derived from oxygen and food).

In a healthy state, the vast majority of the body's energy is allocated toward growth, maintenance, and repair. As biological entities age or encounter chronic stress, their action efficiency declines. They lose the ability to maintain their far-from-equilibrium state. When this occurs, the organism's capacity to maintain its far-from-equilibrium order begins to fail. This failure can manifest in either direction: as rising internal noise and structural breakdown, sliding the system toward chaotic, maximum-entropy dissolution, or as a rigid over-constraint that strips the system of the adaptive variability it needs to respond to new demands. It is the former — the noisy, chaotic, inflammatory slide toward entropic collapse — which this essay is concerned with.

Inflammation is fundamentally the body's localized, protective mechanism to maintain its integrity in response to macroscopic or microscopic injuries, whether physical, environmental, or psychological. However, a vigorous, multipronged, chronic inflammatory response operates at an exceedingly high metabolic cost.

"It is not stress that kills us, it is our reaction to it."
Hans Selye

When an individual experiences prolonged psychosocial stress, physical trauma, or metabolic dysfunction, the brain-body control network enters a state of persistent allostatic accommodation. To fuel this constant state of alert, the organism experiences hypermetabolism, an excess energy expenditure far above its optimum. This added energetic burden is known as the allostatic load. When the chronic energetic cost of stress and low-grade systemic inflammation exceeds the body's reserve capacity, it directly steals energy away from growth, maintenance, and repair processes. From a thermodynamic perspective, chronic illness and intractable pain are states of uncontrolled internal entropy where the body's energy is entirely consumed by a dysfunctional, looping inflammatory cascade, leaving nothing left to repair the system.

Acupuncture is uniquely suited as a tool of choice because it acts as an informational input that re-establishes systemic order through complexity matching and precise neuro-immune regulation. Acupuncture systematically frees the body's trapped metabolic energy, allowing the organism to reduce its internal entropy, restore its self-organizing efficiency, exit hypermetabolism, and restart the vital programs of cellular maintenance, repair, and long-term health. Among the most powerful systemic anti-inflammatory mechanisms of acupuncture is its ability to modulate the vagal-adrenal axis and activate the cholinergic anti-inflammatory pathway. By doing this, acupuncture can interrupt an out-of-control inflammatory response and bring the system back towards a lower-entropy homeostasis setting.

Complexity

"Nature uses only the longest threads to weave her patterns, so that each small piece of her fabric reveals the organization of the entire tapestry."
Richard Feynman

An acupuncture point is not a simple coordinate on the skin; it is a dense, highly complex neurovascular and fascial crossroads, like a vortex of physiological activity. It is an intricate matrix of mechanoreceptors, cells, and nerve endings embedded within a fractal collagen web.

In a healthy state, the time-series data of our vital signs, such as heartbeat intervals, breathing cadences, and neural firing frequencies, are neither completely predictable (like a clock) nor completely random (like white noise). Instead, they display a highly specific mathematical property known as 1/f variability or fractal 'pink noise'. "Pink noise serves as an adequate model for many biological systems and psychological states... deviations from the $1/f$ structure can serve as indicators for disease severity."[1]

This fractal scaling indicates that the human body is a self-organizing, interconnected web. Every organ system continuously exchanges information with every other organ across multiple nested time scales. This structural and temporal elasticity gives a healthy organism its resilience and the ability to dynamically adjust its internal terrain to adapt to unpredictable environmental demands.

Acupuncture utilizes this cross-scale informational exchange to trigger specific neuro-immune resets. When an acupuncturist inserts a needle and the Qi arrives, the manual manipulation generates a complex, multi-scale mechanical and electrical wave. This microcosmic input directly mirrors the fractal dynamics of a healthy nervous system.

When two complex networks interact, information flows from the system with the higher structural and temporal complexity to the system with lower complexity. This phenomenon is known as complexity matching.[2] It is a theory which may help to explain how microcosmic patterning restores macrocosmic patterning through dynamic resonance. We can consider the stimulus at the acupoint to possess a rich, healthy complexity signature, and the systemic, diseased body network may automatically tune itself to this therapeutic input. Stated differently, the broken, low-complexity network of the patient responds to the high-complexity signature of the needling intervention. Perhaps this complexity science theory can help to explain part of the subtlety and wondrousness of acupuncture.

---

1. Measuring Fractality.
2. Complexity Synchronization of Organ Network.

The Unified Empire

"The true lord lives in emptiness, holds fast to the unadorned, and appears to understand nothing; therefore he is able to employ the knowledge of the many. He is wise but has no abilities; therefore he can employ the abilities of the many. He is able to hold fast to doing nothing; therefore he is able to employ the actions of the many. Understanding nothing, being able at nothing, and doing nothing are principles to which a lord holds firm".
The Annals of Lü Buwei, Book 25 Chapter 4.1

Chinese medicine is one of the earliest forms of 'systems physiology'. Not only did the naturalists map the geophysical features of the earth onto human anatomy, with channels as rivers and flesh as earth, they also transferred the terminology of the state's bureaucracy directly onto human physiology.

The relationships between the Emperor (Heart) and its ministers mirror an idealized administrative hierarchy. The Emperor rules supremely but relies entirely on the Prime Minister (Lungs) to transmit decrees, the General (Liver) for defense and strategy, and the Granary Officials (Spleen and Stomach) to sustain the 'bodily population'. The health of the human organism depends on a regular and balanced input of resources, unobstructed transportation channels, adequate storage in the depots, and moderate consumption in the palaces.

If the ministers fulfill their specific duties without obstruction or depletion, the cosmic empire remains peaceful and harmonious. Consequently, illness is conceptualized not merely as a biological failure, but as an administrative breakdown or social chaos within the state. It is the inner version of an empire at risk of collapse, whether from internal threats of rebellion or by external threats of invaders.

The Heart mirrors the sage-king by simply occupying the position of superior and nurturing its spirit. Because the Heart remains a tranquil, central seat of spirit brilliance, it provides the enlightened awareness necessary for the other organs like the Liver (the General) or the Kidneys (the Operator with Force) to exhaust their arts and use all their abilities for the good of the whole system. If the Heart (or the Emperor) were to toil with their bodies, tax their minds, or wear out their senses by trying to micromanage every function, the entire imperial structure of the body would fall into chaos. Perhaps this is a way to understand chronic anxiety — an emperor who cannot help but micromanage and fret over every minister and department of the empire, rather than rely on the skills of each and by doing so remain in stillness and strength, allowing things to take their natural course.

This is just an example of how the political and administrative philosophies of ancient China are imbued within the writings and paradigm of the medicine. Most acupuncturists never study this substrate directly, though, and I think that's a real gap. It isn't decorative background material — it informs the actual logic which the medicine was built from, and without it, concepts such as the organ-official correspondences can start to feel like an arbitrary list to memorize rather than the coherent system they actually are.

Principle

Lǐ 理

All things under heaven can be understood in the light of their principle."
Cheng Yi

Li, translated as principle, order, pattern, or reason, is one of the most fundamental concepts in Chinese philosophy. Its etymology contains the grain found in the cutting of jade, but it evolved into a comprehensive metaphysical category: the inherent order, reason, and moral law that makes each thing what it is. Li is not a physical substance; it is the organizing principle that gives matter its structure, form, and functional meaning. Li is the blueprint of the Dao. It is the reason a snowflake forms a fractal hexagon, why rivers branch into deltas, and why blood vessels mirror the branching of trees. In essence, it is the grain of reality.

A core axiom of classical Chinese cosmology is that the human body is a microcosm that perfectly mirrors the macrocosm of the universe. When we say microcosmic Li restores macrocosmic Li, we are invoking a holographic paradigm. In a true hologram, the whole is not merely the sum of its parts; rather, every individual part contains the structural information of the entire whole.

An acupuncture point is a localized node of supreme microcosmic Li. It represents an instance of the body's original organizational blueprint. When a needle is inserted into an active point and the Qi arrives, we are essentially striking a tuning fork at a node of microcosmic Li. Acting as a conduit between the macro and microcosms, acupuncture's input alters the entire fractal holographic matrix. This principle exists independent of us. The needle does not impose order on the body any more than the jade-carver's blade imposes the grain which it follows. It simply reveals a pattern that was already there and taps into a pre-existing blueprint of the body.

The Cellular Crystalline Axis

"The twelve primary conduits are like the great rivers... The Eight Extra-ordinary Meridians act as ditches, lakes, and reservoirs."
The Classic of Difficult Issues

The eight extraordinary vessels reach back to the moment of conception, the 'big bang' of our own life. The moment the sperm fertilizes the egg, the primordial Source Qi ignites at what becomes the *mingmen* or Gate of Life. The very first division of cells establishes the Chong Mai (Thoroughfare Vessel), traditionally called the 'Sea of Blood' and the 'Ancestor of the twelve Channels'. The Chong Mai is the central axis of cellular proliferation, it serves as the sea of the twelve channels.

"If there is one evolutionary source (Kidney Jing) from which the three vessels emerge, i.e., the Ren, Du and Chong Mai, then the Chong Mai can be seen as the most vital interface supporting and connecting the three axes of development."
Kiiko Matsumoto

From this axis, the embryo undergoes polarization, splitting into an anterior-posterior and dorsal-ventral orientation — Yin and Yang:

"The Conception and Governing vessels are like midnight and midday, they are the polar axis of the body ... there is one source and two branches, one goes to the front and the other to the back of the body ... When we try to divide

these, we see that yin and yang are inseparable."
Li Shi-zhen[1]

- The Du Mai (Governing Vessel) emerges on the dorsal aspect, guiding the formation of the neural tube, the spinal cord, and the central nervous system from the primitive streak.

- The Ren Mai (Conception Vessel) emerges on the ventral aspect, guiding the midline creation of the digestive tube, the thoracic cavity, and the structural front of the body.

"The Yàng Heel, the Yàng Tie, together with the Governing and Belt [extraordinary vessels], master diseases of the shoulder, back, waist, and legs located exteriorly."
The Ode of Mysterious Indications, from the Zhenjiu Dacheng

As the embryo rapidly expands, it faces a massive thermodynamic challenge: it must prevent its own growth from scattering into chaotic randomness, so it needs boundaries.

- The Dai Mai (Girdling Vessel) binds the horizontal axis. It acts like a belt, wrapping around the waist line to hold the vertical expansion of the Chong, Du, and Ren vessels in a tight, coherent geometric grip.

- The Yin and Yang Qiao Mai (Heel Vessels) manage the left-right spatial balance and structural symmetry, ensuring that the limbs and eyes develop with perfect, mirrored proportion.

- The Yin and Yang Wei Mai (Linking Vessels) act as the temporal and spatial connective framework, linking the deep internal Zang layers to the superficial Fu layers as the tissues differentiate.

"The Yīn Heel, the Yīn Tie, the Conception and the Thoroughfare vessels, remove illnesses of the Heart, abdomen, flanks and ribs located interiorly

which are uncertain or persistent."
The Ode of Mysterious Indications, from the Zhenjiu Dacheng

The eight extraordinary vessels serve as the embryological scaffolding. They are the primordial closure of constraints for the morphogenetic field, an overarching, spatial-temporal blueprint that coordinates cellular behavior across an embryo.

"The dynamic Qi that moves between the Kidneys is [the basis] of human life, the source of the five zang and six fu, the root of the twelve channels, the door of respiration and the origin of the sanjiao."
Nan Jing, Chapter 8

As the embryo divides along its initial polarized axis, it follows recursive, self-similar rules: branch, grow, and repeat. This embryological development, guided by the energetic template of the cellular axis, embodies the universal scaling laws that govern human anatomy. Hierarchical, fractal-like distribution networks maximize the surface area available for resource exchange (i.e., capillaries, cell membranes, mitochondria) while minimizing internal transport distances and times, optimizing the body's energetic efficiency and displaying the grand miracle of our biological design.

But when we are fully formed, the extraordinary vessels do not just disappear; they recede into the deep background of our physiology. They are the archetypes of the original principle or pattern, and they remain permanently connected to the deepest, most foundational reserves of the body: the marrow, the bones, the brain, and the Kidney essence. During daily life, if a patient experiences a massive shock, a violent external pathogen, or a raging storm of chronic systemic inflammation, the twelve primary rivers can overflow, unable to handle the entropic overload. The body dumps this excess pathogenic noise and heat into the extraordinary reservoirs to protect the vulnerable organs.

This reveals that the master and coupled point pairs of the eight extraordinary vessels are not just arbitrary points, but are in fact critical transmission nodes designed to recalibrate the body's multi-scale fractal architecture by tapping into the body's deepest embryological reservoirs. The master and couple points for the extraordinary vessels are some of the most potent points available in the clinic.

---

1. Manual of Acupuncture.

Regulation

Tiáo 調

"It is stated that, in the administration of acupuncture, the knowledge of how to regulate (Yin and Yang) is essential. Once yin and yang are well regulated, the essential Qi is bountiful, form and Qi are united, and the spirit is stored in the interior."
The Systematic Classic of Acupuncture and Moxibustion

Tiao means 'to regulate, to adjust, or to tune.' It is the active, pragmatic process by which harmony is reached and maintained. If harmony is the destination, regulation is the vehicle to get there. The universe, the state, and the body are all dynamic entities; continuously shifting systems of Qi. Harmony is therefore never a static achievement but a dynamic state which requires continuous, attentive regulation to be maintained.

"'To regulate' means to put into order. It is said that the needle can regulate and treat illnesses of the viscera and bowels. If there is cold then warm it, if there is heat then purge it, if there is deficiency then supplement it, if there is excessive tension or obstructive blockage then dispel it by expelling the eight evils."
The Ode of Mysterious Indications, from the Zhenjiu Dacheng

In this sense, acupuncture is the art of tuning the Qi of the body with the needle. Much like adjusting the strings of an instrument allows it to play in harmony, the effects of acupuncture tune the Qi of the body. Health is then conceived as a state of perfect internal tuning. Disease is therefore its opposite, manifesting in excesses or deficiencies, disharmonies and dysregulations. This also extends beyond the physical to the mental-emotional realm and the balancing of one's internal desires.

> *"A person's whole body is just like Heaven and Earth. The Qì of Heaven and Earth does not have the means to be in constant obeyance and must await the merits of patterning and bounding. The Qì of the body does not have the means to be in constant balance and must await the techniques of regulation and nurturing."*
> *Yang Jizhou, Essay on the Gains and Losses of the Various Schools, from the Zhenjiu Dacheng*

Furthermore, since a living being is such a dynamic entity in a continuous state of change, interfacing with environments which can be injurious or even hostile, there are times when disharmony or chaos is perhaps inevitable. Even in the natural world there are instances when severe excesses and deficiencies occur. We might think of devastating droughts, intense storms, or chaotic floods. In these cases, acupuncture exists as a tool to retune the body's Qi back to a state of harmony by regulating and nurturing it, steering it away from the extremes of excess or deficiency.

Prevention

"An ounce of prevention is worth a pound of cure."
Benjamin Franklin

Preventing problems before they arise falls squarely into the category of common sense. Anyone can clearly see this, and yet we find that it is rarely practiced. Patients often come to us when they already have problems which they need to address, or after they have been through the healthcare mill, seeking us out in desperation and having exhausted their options; but in the course of solving their issues we have the opportunity to educate them with a beneficial philosophy and help them to internalize it.

"The superior technique is used to prevent disease, not to cure what is already diseased."
Ling Shu, Chapter 55

It is a common motif in the Chinese classics to emphasize the importance of prevention rather than treatment. Harmonious living is their preferred prescription in order to never fall ill in the first place. Understanding one's place in the cosmos and one's environment and living according to the natural fluctuations of Qi is the essence of this lifestyle. Eating, drinking, and acting in a proper manner, avoiding excess or deficiency. Cultivating and nourishing health, rather than treating disease. Being proactive is valued higher than reactivity. Fixing a problem is good, but what about never having it in the first place? I believe in the idea that maintenance is always better, easier, and cheaper than repair.

> *"Prevent trouble before it arises. Put things in order before they exist. The giant pine tree grows from a tiny sprout. The journey of a thousand miles starts from beneath your feet."*
> *Dao De Jing, Chapter 64*

Yet of course in life it is possible for problems to occur and to find us, even if we exercise prudence. Catching a problem early is essential so that it does not grow into something unmanageable. Keen observation and awareness can assist in identifying an emerging issue before it takes root. Perhaps it begins as simply as an inappropriate habit or an unhealthy pattern of thinking. One reason it is important to communicate and build rapport is so that we may gain insights into our patient's lives and habits. The longer an issue persists, the deeper it penetrates, and the more problematic and difficult to remove it becomes. Soon the tiny sprout becomes a large tree. If we can see the propensity for where things will lead, we can intervene before they manifest and actualize.

> *"The fact is, when a disease persists over a long time, it is transmitted in the organism and it is transformed."*
> *Su Wen, Chapter 3*

The classics paint a picture of an idyllic time when the ancients lived in harmony with the world. For them medicine was less important because they cultivated their Qi, practiced Qigong and Daoyin, breathwork, imbibed life-nourishing herbs, prevented illness by protecting their bodies, spirits, and their essence. They ate and drank appropriately and accorded their behavior to the seasons. Thus they were able to quickly bring any emerging diseases to an end before they had a chance to begin.

> *"In this peaceful and tranquil world, the evil was unable to penetrate deeply."*
> *Su Wen, Chapter 13*

Neuroplasticity

Neuroplasticity is the nervous system's capacity to physically remodel its own circuits in response to experiences. It is one of the most important mechanisms to understand how acupuncture's local mechanical signals become a durable, system-wide reset rather than a temporary symptom mask.

Our nervous systems are highly adaptive. Chronic or overwhelming stress, for instance, engages the same neural remodeling machinery in a maladaptive way. The structure and connectivity of our brains mirror these chronic or acute stress states. Chronic pain is another example — sustained pain inputs will increase central nervous system excitability. Over time, these types of chronic input will 'weather' the brain, shrinking regions like the prefrontal cortex and disrupting the Default Mode Network (DMN), conforming the nervous system to rigid, pathological configurations. But this neuroplastic effect goes both ways. We are also capable of changing these configurations in a positive sense, and this is where acupuncture comes in as a useful means to this end.

When needle manipulation produces the De Qi sensation, it triggers a complex neural response. For example, De Qi initiates a coordinated deactivation of the Limbic-Paralimbic-Neocortical Network, modulating and even reversing the pathological connectivity patterns seen in chronic pain, depression, and allostatic load.[1] DMN deactivation could be considered a Yin neural state, while task-positive activation is Yang. Acupuncture also causes the release of an array of neurotransmitters, such as opioids, adenosine, serotonin, acetylcholine, and others. These signaling molecules induce potent effects on the nervous system, spurring neuroplastic responses. The brain actually rewires its connections in response to acupuncture treatment. This is partially why acupuncture's effects persist over time, rather than simply mask symptoms. It is also a strong argument for *regular* acupuncture as a practice, in order to repeatedly reinforce its effects. Explaining these elements of acupuncture to a patient can help them to understand the nature of its effects in a language which is familiar to them.

Because network-level neuroplasticity is systemic rather than single-target, it offers a robust mechanism for acupuncture succeeding where single-target drugs fail on self-reinforcing chronic-disease loops. This is one of the powerful and unique features of acupuncture, and it is emblematic of its holistic nature. In a world where complex, multi-system chronic diseases are so prevalent and on the rise, acupuncture stands as a potent tool and practice which can be leveraged to make lasting neuroplastic changes.

---

1. Acupuncture, the limbic system, and the anticorrelated networks of the brain.

Internal Essays

The essays in this section pertain to topics related to the practitioner's behavior, their inner condition. These essays feel softer, more philosophical or internal; things such as mental-emotional states, dispositions, or relationships. I think of these as the Yin essays of the book. These essays are more poetic, philosophical, and personal to me. They are less about established theory or practice and more about my personal sentiments regarding different aspects of the experience of being an acupuncturist, and ways of being which I find useful.

Spirit

"One must be one unity with the spirit. This is the will of the needle."[1]
Ling Shu, Chapter 3 and Su Wen, Chapter 54

According to the classics, the Spirit is perhaps the most essential aspect of acupuncture. Calmness and clarity of the mind is sharper than the tip of a needle. A dull Spirit will make one's treatments equally dull. To treat without being rooted in Spirit can even cause harm as it is wayward and lost in its action.

"All norms of piercing require one to first of all consider the spirit as the foundation."
Ling Shu, Chapter 8

Spirit is the result of the mutual interactions of Yin and Yang. Spirit is rooted in the harmonious interplay of the Blood and Qi, the substance and function of our being. The Spirit is preserved and flourishes when Yin and Yang are in harmony. Excessive indulgence of desires, stressors, or emotional disturbances harm the Qi and creates imbalance in our physiological homeostasis. Therefore, to live in harmony with the internal and external world is to nourish life. This is essential practice for the practitioner. To be effective, our Spirit must be harmonious.

"With the Spirit, anything that is sought can be found, and anything that is done can be accomplished."
Wen Zi, Chapter 31

Now in acupuncture, the Spirit of the patient must also be attended to and the condition of their Spirit must be appraised in diagnosis. This is why we inspect the Qi, its comings and goings, and attempt to understand the balance of Yin and Yang and the state of the organs and bodily systems. According to the *Ling Shu*, the first principle of acupuncture is to regulate the Spirit, as it is the foundation.[2] "Unrefined [practitioners] guard the physical appearance. Outstanding [practitioners] guard the spirit."[3] With our own Spirit calm, centered, and unconfused, we apply the acupuncture according to our diagnosis. If the Qi arrives and harmony is reestablished, the Spirit will return and disharmony will be regulated.

> *"Close the door and shut the windows, tie yourself to the patient, repeatedly inquire about their feelings, adapt your treatment to their sentiments. If one gets ahold of the spirit, the patient will prosper; if the spirit is lost, the patient perishes."*
> *Su Wen, Chapter 13*

---

1. This quote combines elements of both chapters.

2. Ling Shu, Chapter 8

3. Ling Shu, Chapter 1

Self Cultivation

"To cure people is to cure the self. To cure that is to cure this. To cure the small is to cure the great. To cure the state is to cure the household. When we are without rebellion, then we are able to cure, for when things are smooth and flowing, they are complete."
Ling Shu, Chapter 29

Being an effective acupuncturist is downstream of one's own self cultivation. It is a function of all of the time and effort spent learning and practicing through one's lifetime; increasing one's knowledge and expertise, growing one's wisdom and life experience. It is a lifelong process of accumulation, refinement, and growth. Spending the time, energy, and effort on self-cultivation will ultimately and fundamentally determine one's depth of practice of the art of acupuncture, just like anything else in life.

Self cultivation is an important aspect of Confucian philosophy. It is an ethical imperative to become the best version of ourselves possible as this results in the greatest benefit to society as a whole and fulfills our ethical obligation to humanity by being an 'upright', *Zhèng* human being. As acupuncturists, it is an added ethical imperative in the sense that we will have the greatest success in treating our patients if we have put the utmost effort into attempting to perfect our art and ourselves.

"Human beings are similar in their natural tendencies, but vary greatly by virtue of their habits."
Analects of Confucius, 17.2

To continually practice and give our energy to self cultivation is to manifest the greatest expression of our latent individual potential into the world. As humans, it is to become our truest selves. As acupuncturists, self cultivation leads to the greatest flowering of our medical art. In my opinion, this ongoing *purposeful striving* towards mastery is what separates a good practitioner from becoming a great one. The masters of all art forms dedicate their lives to their art.

Practice

"We are what we repeatedly do. Excellence, then, is not an act, but a habit."
Will Durant

Practice is central to self cultivation, growth, and the development of human beings. This of course applies to acupuncturists as well. Human beings are essentially practicing creatures; humans are like 'people in training'. Even if we are not consciously aware that it is happening, we are continually undergoing a process of self transformation through practice. In this sense, the human being is that which struggles against itself continually in order to form itself.

It is important to discern useful practices from harmful ones. We must consciously choose the practices which will send us in the ideal developmental directions. We must also weed out unconscious practices which are impressed upon us by outside forces. In all likelihood, those unconscious practices do not have the best interests of our self development at their basis. "There are only regimens that are more and less capable and worthy of propagation."[1] Particularly for niche or specialty arts, of which acupuncture is definitely a unique and unorthodox one (at least in the modern *western* world), specialized and often eccentric practices are required.

As acupuncturists, what practices are beneficial to us? Anything which aims to improve our capabilities and capacities as acupuncture practitioners. Anything which pulls us towards greater vertical heights in our art form. We must develop acupuncture practice regimens for ourselves and continually refine our practice. "Practice is defined here as any operation that provides or improves the actor's qualification for the next performance of the same operation, whether it is declared as practice or not."[2]

Every time we enter the clinic is an opportunity to engage in acupuncture specific practices — use the sensitivity of our hands, practice diagnosis skills, or refine our needling techniques. But even outside of the clinic we have numerous opportunities. Each time we read a book or open up a classic, engage in philosophy, study a new subject, or learn a new technique, we are practicing. Even physical exercise, meditation, Qi Gong, diet, and other techniques; anything which helps us function at a higher level as acupuncturists can be considered part of the amalgamation of our practice regiments. Embodying the Taoist principles and philosophy which underlies acupuncture by simplifying and harmonizing our lives might be a starting point.

There are many forces competing for our attention and practice these days. Finding opportunities to switch the phone out for a book goes a long way over a long time horizon. Little practices and modifications of our habits add up if done consistently and consciously over time. We have three options for how to be when it comes to practice: we can choose "between the practicing and the untrained, or *those who train differently*."[3]

---

1. You Must Change Your Life
2. Ibid.
3. Ibid.

Habits

"Our character is basically a composite of our habits. Because they are consistent, often unconscious patterns, they constantly, daily, express our character."
Stephen R. Covey

The human being is not a finished product but an ongoing project. In East Asian philosophy, there is a core belief that anyone can become a sage through deliberate, lifelong character development, a process of self-cultivation. This frames our life as an ongoing process of *becoming*, of transformation, and this is achieved in principle through our practices and our habits. We as humans are in a relationship with ourselves whereby we 'work on ourselves' to facilitate change, growth, and development. Every operation or action performed inevitably reacts upon the actor, meaning that the worker is intimately shaped by their work, the thinker by their thoughts, and the feeler by their feelings.

This leads directly to the concept of the practicing human, or the human in training. A 'human in training' is an individual who embraces the practicing life, struggling with their own form and consciously responding to the ethical imperative to establish new, higher-level habits through disciplined routines. In any specialized field or craft, of which acupuncture is certainly one, these principles act as the foundational mechanisms for achieving mastery and virtuosity. The true core of craftsmanship lies in the convergence of production and practice.[1]

"Nothing is stronger than habit."
Ovid

An acupuncturist treating a patient is simultaneously operating on themselves, shaping their own identity, focus, and mastery through the act of healing others. The time they spend studying the classics, reading the works of the great masters before them, and refining their craft, feeds back into every future moment of their practice. Once the acupuncturist has built a massive foundation through thousands of hours of practice and study, they can creatively and intuitively adapt to the improbable situations of each unique patient, acting perfectly in the spirit of the exact right moment.

The development of a craft, therefore, is not merely about producing an external product, but is an ongoing, self-referential project of sculpting the creator's own human potential and biological capacities through disciplined training. So my challenge to you is to develop your own practice regimens, to struggle to form yourself towards an ideal of acupuncture self-mastery. As Nietzsche would say, to "take yourself in hand!"

---

1. Sloterdijk, P. You Must Change Your Life.

Vertical Tension

"Excellence is difficult, but to be mediocre is no pressure."
Kat Williams

What drives us? What brings us to strive for greater mastery, skill, and proficiency in our trade? Left to the devices of inertia, humans can fall victim to unconscious habits, bad practices, and become formed in ways which do not serve this greater purpose. The ideal to become virtuosic at our craft is very specific and requires conscious efforts, programmed habits, and practices which serve our ends. It involves actively assuming responsibility for one's own life, values, and destiny, rather than passively accepting external influences or conforming to societal norms. In essence, this is a form of self-reliance.

One way to orient ourselves is to establish this ideal as our vertical tension. This is a concept which describes the inescapable human drive to elevate oneself, improve, and reach higher states of achievement or being.[1] It operates along an inner vertical axis that establishes a polarity between above and below in any given field, such as the contrast between excellence and mediocrity, knowledge and ignorance, or perfection and incompletion. This tension acts as a magnetic pull or attractor from a higher pole, compelling individuals to evaluate their current, flawed state against a superior ideal. By consciously establishing this vertical tension we establish the conditions to pull ourselves upwards towards our ideal.

"Craftsmanship names an enduring, basic human impulse, the desire to do a job well for its own sake."
Richard Sennett

The craftsman is fundamentally quality-driven, propelled by an obsessional energy to do good work for its own sake rather than merely achieving a minimum standard. The vertical ascent in a trade begins with brute imitation of the master's procedures. However, as the practitioner climbs higher, the goal shifts from copying to achieving true autonomy. The ultimate expression of overcoming vertical tension is when the practitioner no longer has to consciously think about the mechanics of their tools or hands; their highly trained body acts intuitively, anticipating problems and adapting to unique situations seamlessly.

> *"Each time one opens up the text and takes counsel in its methods, page by page, carefully investigate its aims. Return to press the classics and examine their words, character by character, their merits are clearly understood. All hidden doubts are known. What is true or false is completely grasped. Removing aches and stopping pain as if by a spirit, below the needle, one obtains peace."*
> *Ode Pointing to the Subtleties of the Ebb and Flow, from Zhenjiu Dacheng*

---

1. Sloterdijk, P. You Must Change Your Life.

Medical Reality

Reality is downstream of politics, economics, culture, and ideology. These are ultimately the powerful forces which shape medicine. We should examine the forces which shape medicinal sociorealities[1] today and question whatever is presented to us as orthodox or reflexively true. Apply skepticism to everything. Every age, every culture, every society, every tradition, has embodied a different reality during the course of time. Each reality brings fresh insights, strengths, weaknesses. They all present us with something valuable to consider. Each way of seeing the world is like a double-edged sword, simultaneously illuminating and occluding.

Ultimately, no representation of reality formulated by humans can yet be said to be completely accurate. If it was, then the problems of medicine, disease, and health would be solved. We should keep this in mind when we are presented with a reality which claims to offer Absolute Truth. Care must be taken not to confuse lower-case reality with upper-case Reality, which exists independently of us and is likely outside of our full ability to apprehend it.

Medical reality has always been pluralistic, even though it is continuously under immense pressure by reality-structuring forces mentioned above. It is shaped by the contributions of many different individuals and systems of thought, each offering shifting realities throughout time. Each reality has enriched the body of medical knowledge with its own ideas of how things are. We can learn from old ideas, and we can learn from new ideas. We can choose to see things in different ways, and hold different realities at the same time. Ideas which seem outdated can provide fresh insights, while ideas which are new can seem useful or exciting, but end up lacking. Investigating history exposes us to these shifting currents of thought.

Learning to hold realities without strictly identifying with them is useful. The more realities we can hold without becoming attached or overly identified, the more flexible and creative we can be with applying a multitude of different ideas towards complex problems.

Perhaps this approach of holding a composite of opposing or even conflicting ideas at the same time can bring us closer to Reality as such.

---

1. Medicine in China: A History of Ideas

Pluralism

The history of medicine spans back to beyond the beginnings of human civilization. In China, there is a written record which reaches thousands of years to the earliest recorded dynasties. Throughout the development and evolution of medicine, ideas concerning health, disease, and medicine shifted radically as society fundamentally altered its paradigmatic realities alongside the rise and fall of political, economic, social, and ideological regimes. Rather uniquely, Chinese medicine retained a pluralistic attitude towards these ideas through time.[1]

Today, we receive this unbroken thread of medical evolution within the context of our own modern socioreality and paradigm. We have the unique opportunity to study and apply ideas and concepts from time periods and contexts worlds apart from our contemporary reality. This plurality and coexistence of ideas is potent because it offers different, unique perspectives to problems. We should strive to retain the essence of the various historical sociorealities and medical paradigms of thought which have been preserved and handed down to us. By doing this, we nurture a broader, fuller, more robust collection of reality lenses through which we can view a problem and devise a novel solution.

Powerful new insights can be discovered from the interplay between ideas, such as ancient and modern. Like a static effect, rubbing together distinctive paradigms of thought can yield sparks. It is like the smashing of atoms together; unanticipated reactions and combinations can occur. While purists seek to keep ideas from touching, comparative philosophy breeds new forms and fresh lines of flight[2] for thought to take.

Our contemporary moment holds vast potential as the most powerful thought paradigms crash into and intermix with one another. We have yet to witness the full results of western science and modern biomedicine's chemical reaction upon meeting the ancient eastern medical realities and traditions, which include acupuncture, herbal medicine, and the philosophies of the east. It is akin to tectonic plates pushing towards one another, forming entirely new mountain ranges. We have the opportunity to explore these fertile, comparative, pluralistic territories as pioneers and explorers.

---

1. Medicine in China: A History of Ideas

2. A Thousand Plateaus.

Syncretism

Syncretism refers to the combining of different forms of belief or practice.[1] Acupuncture, as part of the vast pluralism of Chinese medicine, is at its heart syncretic. Acupuncture theory and practice in general has been influenced throughout the millennia by many different thinkers, books, systems, and schools of thought.

It is a human tendency to always want to identify and put a label onto something. Humans like when things are put into their separate, clearly labelled boxes. They like when systems of thought are clearly delineated, and when forms of practice are divided by clear lines. This provides a simplified and inaccurate convenience. Particularly today there is a reductionist proclivity in medicine. But reality is more complex, colors bleed over the lines, and systems of thought and practice intermix and form unorthodox blends. Even ideas which seem opposite can become combined and emulsified, much like Yin and Yang.

The complexity of medicine has inspired a panoply of manifestations of how one practices acupuncture. Each practitioner takes influence from a variety of sources and individualizes themselves by their unique process of practice and accumulated experience. This creates a syncretic form of acupuncture that is quintessentially their own; it is a reflection of themselves and their art form. This is the nature of art. Over time we learn new ideas, are introduced to new schools of thought, put new concepts into practice, and master new skills. Embracing syncretism means we strive to have as many useful tools in our acupuncture toolbox as possible in order to meet the demands of medicine. There is no school of thought which can claim to be perfect or to have all of the answers, although many often do claim to.

The philosophical underpinnings of acupuncture spring from syncretic soils. It has always been the case, since the beginnings of Chinese culture, that competing ideas, systems of thought, and ways of seeing the world mutually coexisted and influenced one another. This can be traced back to the Warring States period and the Hundred Schools of Thought, which saw the flourishing of competing philosophies as well as in medicine, which was imbued with the syncretism of Huang-Lao thought and the classics during the Han Dynasty. Likewise, during the Song-Jin-Yuan era, a multitude of new schools emerged, each with unique contributions and ideologies. These periods of development were pivotal to the development of East Asian medicine.

Today we stand on a new precipice where East meets West. We have the opportunity to enrich our practice with an even more pluralistic and syncretic blend of influences which spans back to ancient times while also including modern forms as well. What novel forms of practice might emerge from this great event?

---

1. Merriam-Webster Dictionary.

Love of Learning

Hàoxué 好學

"Reviewing the old as a means of realizing the new – such a person can be considered a teacher."
Analects of Confucius, 2.11

Confucius' 'love of learning' suggests a continuous, life-long, enthusiastic pursuit of knowledge, not just for knowledge's sake but for moral improvement and social harmony. In the context of medicine, embodying this attitude toward learning may yield the best results for our patients because as acupuncturists we will be in a position to use our acquired knowledge in order to assist them in their medical needs. Could it even be said that there is an *ethical imperative* for us to do so as we assume this important role and function? In this sense, embodying a love of learning is an essential part of our job as acupuncturists.

"Learning without due reflection leads to perplexity; reflection without learning leads to perilous circumstances."
Analects of Confucius, 2.15

Cultivating a love of learning is thus a moral duty we have in life. To embrace learning is an act of wisdom. Learning is an important component in the act of perfecting our potential and becoming a better, more effective and fully realized version of ourselves. We all owe it not just to ourselves to do this but also to our patients, our ancestors, and to society as a whole. In some ways, this is serious business! To skirt this responsibility could even be somewhat negligent. But ultimately, it is supposed to be fun. Learning feels good; it is the flowering of our potential, the development of our capabilities. It is a sweet, slowly unfolding satisfaction. Love the process!

> *"As a general principle, you must work to progress in your studies; then your heart will not suffer any perplexity."*
> *The Annals of Lü Buwei, Book 4 Chapter 3.3*

Learning Before the Encounter

"From words one can obtain knowledge. From inspection one can obtain insights."
Su Wen, Chapter 39

Diagnosis is a robust process. On one hand it happens in an immediate sense as we inspect the patient and identify signs and patterns of disorder or disruption of harmony. But it also operates on a different dimension with a much longer time scale, as it involves drawing from the accumulated reservoir of knowledge which we acquire over a lifetime of enthusiastic learning and gathering of experience.

In the clinic, we want to be best prepared for whatever we may encounter. The ideal scenario is that we already know how to solve an issue before the patient who has it even walks through our door. We do this by dedicating our time to learning in order to be prepared ahead of time.

The next best scenario is when we encounter a problem, and though we may not have a firm grasp of the solution, we engage with our resources in order to figure out a solution and thus gain experience in the process. This again requires a process of learning, immersing ourselves within the classics, reading the science, experimentation, intuition, and becoming absorbed with whatever other materials we have at our disposal in order to gain an edge and attain a better understanding and method of treatment.

"Remove the old and approach the new. Then you acquire the status of a true human."
Su Wen, Chapter 13

The worst case scenario is when we have a predefined idea about a problem which is wrong but which we nonetheless cling to and try to force to work, refusing to change our methods to adapt to the situation. Instead of a mind which is humble and open, we remain closed with a sense of hubris.

While we may at times fail to solve an issue for a patient, and this is perhaps a necessary part of the learning process for any acupuncturist, the ultimate failure is to not take this lesson to heart or use it as a stimulus to learn, adapt, and prepare for the next time we meet this problem again so that we are better and successful then. Failures are often what lead to later success, but only if we use them properly, as learning instruments.

In this sense, medicine is truly a practice, a continual dialogue, an ongoing development. We must be ready to change our ways of thinking and practicing and remain flexible. Embrace the lifelong learning process of acupuncture; lean into it, and turn it into an aspect of your practice. Embody a robust love of self-directed learning so that we can perform our duties for our patients at the highest possible level.

Remonstrance

Remonstrance is the act of pointing out or opposing something which is wrong or misguided. In Confucianism, remonstrance is a profound moral imperative in hierarchical relationships, particularly those between minister and ruler, or child and parent. Because the health of the state and the family depended on the moral rectitude of its head, subordinates were duty-bound to speak up when their superiors erred. Remonstrance is not an act of defiance, but the ultimate expression of loyalty, filial piety, and love. It was one's duty as a loyal advisor to attempt to avert destruction by remonstrating with the emperor.

> *"In the face of whatever is not right, the son cannot but remonstrate with his father, and the minister cannot but remonstrate with his prince. If it is not right, remonstrate!"*
> *Confucius, The Book of Filial Piety, Chapter 15*

While we today are not within a Confucian hierarchical structure, we might still apply this precept to our relationship with our patients, as we are their minister-advisors. If we fail to speak up to correct harmful actions, or alert our patients to harmful behaviors, habits, and practices, we may be partially to blame in the resulting harm which befalls them. But if we gently remonstrate with them, we fulfill our ethical duties as a medical advisor appropriately.

> *"Good medicine is bitter to the tongue but efficacious in treating illness; loyal speech is offensive to the ear but efficacious in improving behavior".*
> *Confucius in Garden of Eloquence, 9.25*

Just as a loyal minister must remonstrate at the first intimations of destruction, a good physician must alert the patient when an illness is still superficial. This evokes the story of the famous physician Bian Que and Duke Huan of Cai. Bian Que repeatedly warned the Duke that he had a disease in his skin, then his flesh, and then his intestines. Because the "medicinal speech" was offensive to his ears, the Duke ignored the physician, claiming, "Physicians love to take credit for curing people who are not sick!". By ignoring the physician's remonstrance, the disease penetrated to the bone marrow, mirroring a state falling into irreversible chaos.

In counseling a patient we must address the patient's lifestyle and mindset, their desires, anxieties, and lack of moderation, because these are the influences generating the physical illness. And we must use tact, perhaps employing 'indirect admonishment' to guide the patient toward changing their destructive habits (like overeating, drunkenness, or emotional extremes) without provoking defensiveness. Remonstrance does not come from a place of judgment; rather, it is compelled by compassion, benevolence, and humaneness.

Seasons

"There is no season such delight can bring, As summer, autumn, winter and the spring."
William Browne

The yearly seasons represent the fluctuating, cyclical exposure of the Earth to warming Yang Qi of the Sun. The idea that one should live in accordance with the seasons, and with repeating cycles of Qi, is an ancient one. Behavioral adaptation to the environment is necessary to preserve physiological harmony.

"They come to life through the Spring; They grow through the Summer; They are collected through Autumn; They are stored away through Winter."
Su Wen, Chapter 6

Since nature is a fractal, there are time cycles which wax and wane at different speeds. The seasons change over the course of a year, but a single day can be a season, as well as a lunar cycle. An individual's entire life can be viewed in terms of its fluctuating seasons. Indeed, even empires have seasons.

"Seasons are defined by spring's warmth, summer's heat, autumn's coolness, and winter's cold; these are the proper Qì of the four seasons."
The Ode of Mysterious Indications, from the Zhenjiu Dacheng

Even acupuncture treatment can vary according to the season. Because the body's Qi mimics nature, it fluctuates with the weather. This is another expression of the fractal nature of time, the body, nature, and the environment. The *Nan Jing* and the *Ling Shu* dictate that a practitioner should needle specific points during specific seasons to harmonize the microcosm with the macrocosm. A simple guideline for applying this chronobiological outlook is to consider the following points during each of the seasons:

- **Winter:** Needle the Jing-Well points (when Qi is hidden deep within the "wells") or the He-Sea points.
- **Spring:** Needle the Ying-Spring points (when Qi rises and dashes forward).
- **Summer:** Needle the Shu-Stream points.
- **Late Summer:** Needle the Jing-River points.
- **Autumn:** Needle the He-Sea points (or Jing-River points).

"Start work when the season comes, Stop when the season ends. In this way, the strength of the old and weak can be fully developed. And in half the time. Their achievement will be doubled."
The Annals of Lü Buwei, Book 26, Chapter 3

Harmony

Hé 和

"Harmony is like a stew. Water, fire, jerky, mincemeat, salt, and plum vinegar are used to cook fish and meat. These are cooked over firewood. The master chef harmonizes them, evening them out with seasonings, compensating for what is lacking, and diminishing what is too strong. The noble man eats it and calms his heart."
Yan Ying, Zuo Tradition, Zhao 20.8

Harmony is the goal and the objective of acupuncture in general. Harmony is a well-blended mixture of different parts, like a stew that is perfectly seasoned. It is the productive integration of opposites. Yin and Yang when harmonized yield health, and when in chaos and disorder they yield disease.

"Harmony leads to bodily health, abundance, and strength."
Dragon Tiger Tortoise Phoenix Methods, from the Zhenjiu Dacheng

Harmony appears in many forms. For the emotions, harmony occurs when emotions arise in their correct measure and degree. Personal harmony occurs when the mind is calm, and the desires are moderated. Disharmony can be seen in violent swings of emotions and unstable desire, or the emergence of pain, stress, and inflammation.

"The total Way of acupuncture is to harmonize the Qi and then stop."
Ling Shu, Chapter 9

To maintain harmony, an individual can align their lifestyle with external cosmic rhythms of Qi. This means modulating their sleep, diet, and emotional habits and responses. Practices which induce states of tranquility or a flow state like meditation, reading a good book, or playing an instrument, can induce states of harmony. It is different for everyone — for myself, I like to paint, write, and create. For the Daoists, harmony is found in the return to spontaneity and oneness, and by abandoning artificial human constructs. Get out into nature, follow your intuition, do something spontaneous, enter into a flow state. But sometimes if harmony is lost, then individuals need assistance, and there is no better way to assist and support their harmony than acupuncture.

> *"So it is said, the essentials of using the needle lie in knowing how to harmonize Yin and Yang. In harmonizing Yin and Yang, the essence and the Qi will glow with the joining of the physical body and the Qi energy. This will send Spirit to the inner storage chambers. Therefore it is said, the superior doctor balances the Qi."*
> *Ling Shu, Chapter 5*

Governing

Zhì 治

"Bring your mind into a state of quiet, and your Qi into a state of indifference. Follow the spontaneity of things and hold within you no element of ego. Then the empire will be governed."
Zhuangzi, Chapter 11

Isn't it interesting that Zhuangzi's advice for governing the empire also perfectly describes the Way in which one should govern oneself? And incidentally, it also perfectly describes the Spirit which one embodies during the practice of acupuncture. To be in the state of spontaneous adaptability and open potentiality is an optimal condition for practicing an art because it allows for creative inspiration. To be in a state of quietude is an optimal condition for being maximally aware of subtleties. To be in a state of indifference means one can move in any direction and follow intuition.

"The techniques by which one governs the body and the state share the same principles".
The Annals of Lü Buwei, Book 17 Chapter 1.1

In fact, the character *Zhì* has the dual meaning of 'to treat an illness' and 'to govern'. Just as a ruler must reform laws to fit changing times to promote prosperity of the empire and to avoid anarchy or collapse, a doctor must adapt therapies to the shifting nature of a disease. Because ancient Chinese philosophy systematically conceptualized the human body as a microcosm of the imperial state, there was no conceptual or linguistic boundary between political administration and medical healing. In this sense, one could consider the role of the acupuncturist to be a sort of minister who performs statecraft on the empire of the human body. Because the ailments of the body and the state are isomorphic, the physician and the statesman use parallel strategic logic.

> A physician treats a disease by breaking through physiological blockages, just as a sage-king governs a state by elevating honest ministers who "dare to speak honestly and thus break through the blockages and impediments".
> *The Annals of Lü Buwei, Book 20 Chapter 5.1*

Prince Wen Hui's Acupuncturist

Prince Wen Hui's acupuncturist was treating a patient.

His hands could be seen gently ascertaining the Qi at the wrist with deep intention.

His spirit was fully absorbed and his senses were united and focused on every detail.

With precision, he then inserted his needles painlessly but with great effect.

Exerting great care and communicating each step in his procedure to the patient.

Lighting a flame, he effortlessly placed glass fire cups onto their strategic locations.

One could tell that there was a profound harmony achieved.

"Excellent job!" the Prince commented. "Your method was faultless!"

"Method?" said the acupuncturist.

Laying down his needles, "What I follow is the Dao. It is beyond all methods!"

"When I first began practicing acupuncture I would see the entire patient all at once. In many ways, it was overwhelming. After a few years of gaining experience, it was no longer one big confusion; I began to see important distinctions. But now, I see nothing. My whole being apprehends the Qi. My senses are idle and I allow my Spirit the freedom to work without a predetermined plan, following instinct. I am guided by the natural lines of the channels into the great hollows and cavities of the body; my hands effortlessly locate areas of stagnation and the hidden spaces where the patient's Qi resides."

"A good acupuncturist will use many needles and try different strategies in order to solve a problem. A poor acupuncturist will cover a patient's entire body with needles or use forceful methods, causing great pain – and they may not even have any positive effect! But these days, after so many years, the work is effortless."

"There are subtle holes in the body where the Qi resides; the needle is sharp and keen. When the needle finds those living spaces then the Qi has arrived! Like the flocking of crows or the bite of a fishing rod; a quick flash of lightning! The treatment goes like a breeze."

"True, there are sometimes difficult cases. I can see them coming the moment they arrive at the clinic. So I slow down, observe even more carefully, holding back with meditative patience. And then *zhip! zhip!* – the needles are in and the patient is sleeping."

"I stand still for a few moments and let the joy of the work sink in, cleaning and putting my tools away."

Prince Wen Hui said, "This is it! My acupuncturist has shown me how I ought to live my own life!"[1]

---

1. This is a creative adaptation of the famous story of Prince Wen Hui's butcher, in Chapter 3 of Zhuangzi

Flow

Flow, or the flow state, has been described as the state of optimal experience. Characteristics of flow include a focused concentration on what one is doing in the present moment to the point where action and awareness merge. In the flow state, one may experience the dissolution of the ego or self-consciousness, and the feeling of embodied control within the loss of temporal awareness.[1]

> *"Flow is being completely involved in an activity for its own sake. The ego falls away. Time flies. Every action, movement, and thought follows inevitably from the previous one, like playing jazz."*
> *Mihaly Csikszentmihalyi*

Any artistic and creative craft beckons us to deeply enter into a flow state and acupuncture is no exception. The opportunity to focus single-mindedly on the task at hand is provided with each patient we see. Every clinical encounter is a chance to use our senses to their fullest and to exert our creative intelligence and skills in order to find novel solutions to complex problems. Entering into the acupuncture flow state is optimal practice.

Another sense of flow also involves moving with or against the current of things. Treat in a way which is in accordance with the seasons, with the prevailing Qi of the environment, and with the trend of the illness. If an illness is excessive, drainage is required. If an illness is deficient, then supplementation is needed. Different seasons call for different needling depths. The Qi is located in different regions of the body during the Winter than it is during the Summer, Spring, or Autumn. Our daily actions, too, must accord with the seasonal Qi. A practitioner who is attuned to the flow of Qi works with it rather than against it, foresees problems before they arise, and understands the propensity of an illness.

> "If one acts in accordance with the seasons of heaven, the further development of the disease can be foreseen. Those who act in accordance [with the seasons of heaven], they are the [competent] practitioners. Those who act contrary to them, they are the unrefined ones."
> *Ling Shu, Chapter 44*

This theme of flow resounds throughout ancient Daoist philosophy. To be in harmony with the universe and in resonance with the environment, allowing nature to take its course, we become more of a conduit or transistor for the healing process itself. The division between the self and the needle dissolves. Of the flow state one might ask, 'am I performing this acupuncture, or is the universe performing this acupuncture through me?' By stepping out of the way and going with the flow, we allow the Dao to speak for itself.

> *"The Master allows things to happen. She shapes events as they come. She steps out of the way and lets the Dao speak for itself."*
> *Laozi, Dao De Jing, Chapter 45*

---

1. Investigating the "Flow" Experience: Key Conceptual and Operational Issues

Tranquility

"Quiet peacefulness, absolute emptiness, the true Qi follows these states. When essence and spirit are guarded internally, where could disease come from?"
Su Wen, Chapter 1

In life and acupuncture alike, tranquility—calmness, serenity—nurtures enduring health. A state of tranquility reduces stress and anxiety, fosters emotional balance, and yields a stable, vibrant physiology. Serenity, a spiritual grace, holds inner peace amid life's storms, even as grief stirs beneath its calm. Serenity has been described as "a spiritual quality that involves inner peace despite vicissitudes and even feelings, thus a person can feel grief, yet be serene."[1]

Tranquility applies to the body, the mind, and the emotions. It has been a key focus of many spiritual and mystic traditions for millennia.[2] As with any performance-based practice, tranquility is necessary for the practitioner of acupuncture. A state of tranquility not only heals the patient but also steadies the healer. As in any art of precision, serenity sharpens the acupuncturist's craft. A tranquil mind heightens observation, sparks creative and strategic decisions, and guides steady hands. This results in a better, more focused execution of the craft.

"To feel the movements in the vessels has a Way: emptiness and quietude are to be treasured."
Su Wen, Chapter 17

A quiet, calm mind and demeanor benefits both the diagnostic and treatment process. Without being present, how can one bring full attention to the subtleties of something as refined as pulse diagnosis? If scattered, important details can be missed, forgotten, or easily overlooked. A tranquil mind hones diagnosis. Without a tranquil presence, how can we catch the pulse's subtle movements? Scattered thoughts obscure fine details while tranquility sharpens our blade. This level of focus could be the difference between an optimal or an average acupuncture treatment. Would a samurai want to keep a dull blade?

> *"Do you have the patience to wait till your mud settles and the water is clear?*
> *Can you remain unmoving until the right action arises by itself?"*
> *Dao De Jing, Chapter 15*

Let us follow the advice of Laozi by entering the clinic with a tranquil clarity. Let the muddy thoughts settle and the waters clear before we engage in acupuncture. From this stillness, correct actions flow naturally. From this clarity, the practitioner's true Qi shines forth effortlessly.

---

1. The Brief Serenity Scale: A Psychometric Analysis of a Measure of Spirituality and Well-Being

2. Exploring tranquility: Eastern and Western perspectives

Centered Focus

"When you are calm and stable, careful of attention, the celestial design is always clear, open awareness is unobscured; then you have autonomy in action and can deal with whatever arises."
The Book of Balance and Harmony

An optimal state of mind enables practice at the highest level. This is true for all art forms, and acupuncture is no exception. Acupuncture demands our full presence. From the moment a patient walks through the door we begin the process of observation. We use all of our senses to pick up subtle clues in our effort to craft an accurate diagnosis. This requires careful focus, a centered spirit, keen senses, and an attentive mind.

"The Way of the management of needles is to be focused and centered. One must be tranquil and quiet."
Ling Shu, Chapter 71

After diagnosis comes treatment. It is essential to be centered and focused during the act of needling. We must be aware of many variables when using the needle in order to obtain the optimal results. Needling demands precision—from choosing points to placing and manipulating the needle. Each choice and action hinges on steady intent, tracking the patient's response until the Qi arrives. This requires an extreme level of concentration and focus. We must be attentive to the procedure as well as to the reactions of the patient so that the subtleties do not elude us.

> *"When the Qi has arrived, that is exactly the moment for which one has to be on the alert."*
> *Su Wen, Chapter 27*

Distractions will dull our sensitivity to Qi, make it harder to listen and integrate information, and ultimately reduce the quality of our treatments. Centered focus will help us to perform to the best of our abilities and be conscious of the many variables involved in acupuncture practice, so that we can attain the best results. Let us heed the words of Qi Bo on the importance of being calm and focused:

> *"When the conduit Qi has arrived, guard it carefully lest it is lost. Deep and shallow are at one's mind; far and near are like one. One must be calm as if one looked down into a deep abyss; the hand must be strong as if it held a tiger. The spirit should not be confused by the multitude of things."*
> *Su Wen, Chapter 25*

Scholar-Physicians

Rúyī 儒醫

In the Chinese Confucian tradition, the term *Rú*, often translated as a Confucian or a scholar, refers to individuals who devoted themselves to learning, cultural refinement and the peaceful arts, as opposed to martial prowess.

After Confucianism became the state ideology, the scholars became the administrative backbone of the Chinese empire. Through a rigorous, state-sponsored civil service examination system based on the mastery of classical texts, elite scholars were recruited to fill the ranks of the imperial bureaucracy. It was the highest ideal and goal of the educated to pass the exams and become officials in the service of the emperor. Officials were responsible for the economic, social, ethical, and spiritual welfare of the empire, handling everything from the collection of taxes and the administration of justice to the establishment of education and the promotion of public morality. For some scholars who did not pass the exams, medicine offered a respectable alternative.

Because the human body was conceptualized as a microcosm of the empire, the culture of scholars translated directly into the theory, ethics, and practice of medicine, giving rise to the *Rúyī*, the Scholar-Physician. To be a scholar-physician meant approaching medicine as a classical, textual science. Medical texts like the *Su Wen* explicitly state that judgment and the mind must be based on strict laws and rules; only a practitioner who "follows the classics and observes the calculations" can practice with the due reverence necessary to benefit humanity.[1] This is an ethos which can still be applied today by examining the classics and investigating the root and source of our medical tradition, with powerful results.

A scholar-physician can actively realize the supreme Confucian virtue of humaneness/benevolence by healing the physical sufferings of people, assisting life and nurturing longevity of the populace, thereby fulfilling one's moral duty with practical, compassionate action.

"A man of quality studies widely, fearing only that he will be unable to go over what he has learned. Having gone over what he has learned, he fears only that he will be unable to put it into practice. Having put it into practice, he fears only that he will be unable to use what he has gained to yield to others."

Garden of Eloquence 16.78

---

1. *Su Wen*, Chapter 77

Sage

"Only the sages follow the Way, hence their bodies have no strange diseases."
Su Wen, Chapter 2

The concept of a sage goes back to antiquity in Chinese culture. Sages were thought to be the rare sort of person who embodied moral excellence and were able to achieve a harmonious relationship with the natural principles of the universe. It was considered an ethical and moral ideal to become a person of virtue who lived according to the Way.

"The sages acted on the basis of 'no intervention.' They enjoyed their ability to be peaceful and tranquil. They have followed their desires and their mind was pleased, maintaining absolute emptiness."
Su Wen, Chapter 5

For the Daoists, the sage is someone who embodies stillness within motion; the ability to achieve everything without effort. Unpolished simplicity, spontaneity, and effortless action; a merging of sorts with the cosmic unity of nature. This sort of virtue can be applied to acupuncture by entering into a flow state, following our intuition, and effortlessly responding to each encounter without attachment to the results.

"The transformations of Heaven and Earth are without limit, yet the sage patterns and bounds them so they do not exceed the mean – this is called 'cutting and completing'."
Zhu Xi

For the Confucians, the sage is someone who consciously strives through deliberate effort to bring correctness and benevolence to the human realm. Through their transformative work, they sought to 'pattern and bound' and to regulate and order Yin and Yang and all which would otherwise go to excess or deficiency among Heaven and Earth. In terms of acupuncture, they apply their regulatory techniques to bring excesses and deficiencies back towards the mean. Both of these philosophical approaches differ in their method but align in a goal, which is harmony.

Read Everything

"The reading of all good books is like a conversation with the finest minds of past centuries"
René Descartes

Our medicine is ultimately derived from a culture of books and writing. Books were treasured as vessels of the most important knowledge to be passed down to future generations. When the Emperor of the Qin Dynasty burned the books of competing philosophies, he spared the books on medicine.[1] This is a testament to their immense value and importance to life and society.

The tradition of our medicine is passed down to us through such classic texts. The knowledge of acupuncture is strung together like pearls on a single thread, reaching back eons to the most fundamental classics, like the *Ling Shu*, the *Su Wen* and the *Nan Jing*. The depths, the root, and the heart of this medicine, must be accessed through books. Books are the doorway to the storehouse of knowledge and wisdom. It is through this door that we can enter the Way of the art of acupuncture, and it is through this same door that we can truly engage with and enact the materials which make up the foundation of our practice. Through books, we can have conversations with the greatest medical minds throughout the generations and across cultures, and we can apply their lessons and insights to modern clinical scenarios.

"To learn without tiring is the way to govern oneself. To teach without tiring is the way to govern the people. Few indeed are those who associate with wise teachers and good companions and yet do wrong."
Wen Zi, Chapter 155

We should endeavor to read everything we can about our medicine, from the ancient classics, all the way to the modern present. Why waste time? Read one of the classics. Why be bored? Bring a book to read. When traveling, always have a book along for the ride. And learn how to take detailed notes! Why not make it a fun part of our work to study and read, absorb knowledge, gain experience, and write the lessons down for ourselves? It is like adding manure to soil. Read the things which excite you and you agree with. And also read the things which challenge you and which you may disagree with. Do not limit yourself in your reading, read everything available to be read. This is one of the greatest practices and habits which we can have throughout our lives. We shouldn't squander the opportunity — previous generations did not have the level of access to these books and sources which we enjoy today. Historically, it was often difficult to come into possession of an important book. The main beneficiaries of all of the time we spend reading are ultimately ourselves, but also our patients.

---

1. Records of the Grand Historian.

The Classics

For what are the classics but the noblest recorded thoughts of man? They are the only oracles which are not decayed..."
Henry David Thoreau

We must engage with the classics. They are deep repositories of ancient knowledge. The collective wisdom from ages past. They are like pearls of immense cultural accretion. The entire tree of tradition traces its roots to the classic books. The concepts of medicine come from the seeds of these classics. The classics are the foundation of what we do now in the present.

"To follow the proper Way, I do not forge new paths; with confidence I cherish the ancients."
Confucian Analects, Chapter 7.1

To read the classics is to converse with great people from another age. They passed their experience and knowledge down to us in order to preserve the light of understanding for future generations. We should not let that opportunity go to waste! Their words are immensely valuable and can provide insight into everything we do today. Their thoughts are ancient, yet they represent an entirely fresh perspective to our modern minds. In this way, they are also often timeless.

"A classic is a book that has never finished saying what it has to say."
Italo Calvino

The classics are meant to be read repeatedly. The best books are not intended to only be read just once. Their fullest meaning blossoms like a flower over time. As we ourselves age and gain experience, the inner wisdom of these texts emerge alongside our own evolving understanding. By returning to and rereading them, we allow this process to unfold. Focused, repeated study of the classics is an essential part of learning the art of acupuncture.

> *"Constantly seek out the ancient meanings, because hidden mechanisms exist."*
> *The Ode Pointing to the Subtleties of Ebb and Flow, from the Zhenjiu Da Cheng*

Books are fundamentally at the heart of medicinal and philosophical culture. The written word, the symbolic meaning of each character, transmits deep, condensed layers of meaning and information. Examining and deconstructing each transmission unveils new dimensions to our art form. Every Chinese character is like a fractal which we can enter and explore to uncover deep hidden meanings embedded in the etymology. The choice of each character is imbued with deep purpose. Read that which has been transmitted to us and enact it into practice.

> *"It is necessary to have the light of individual perception and the clarity of individual learning before it is possible to master the Way in action."*
> *Wen Zi, Chapter 160*

Science

Acupuncture, as an ancient art developed many centuries ago, is still quite a mystery to the modern mind. Its inner workings are not yet fully understood by mainstream science. What happens when a fundamental mystery and question arises which meets the inquiry of science?

Whenever something revolutionary meets the orthodox mode of thinking a powerful reaction occurs. Often, the first response is a defensive one, as any revolutionary line of thought is dangerous to the established paradigm which has solidified in place. The kneejerk reaction has been to claim that acupuncture is a pseudoscience and the result of only the placebo effect. This explanation, however, is a shallow way to push aside the uncomfortable questions which the observed effects of acupuncture cause us to ask. As research continues, it becomes apparent that there is much more to acupuncture than placebo alone. The paradoxes of acupuncture research continue to shed light on the pitfalls of contemporary scientific methodologies.[1] It is difficult to casually wave away the virtues of something which has benefitted humanity for many centuries.

I believe that the meeting of acupuncture and science may spark a powerful line of research and a reenergized understanding of human physiology, health, disease, and medicine by initiating a revolution in interconnectedness, integrative philosophy, and holistic thinking. We will be forced to develop new research methodologies and use scientific ingenuity to understand its mysteries. The old methods break down when they are applied to something this complex.

Acupuncture has the potential to break apart the reductionist ideologies which currently have stagnated medicine in our modern world, and this will reshape deep aspects of our modern medical world views. The holistic effects of acupuncture resist the tendencies of modern medicine to create silos and specialties and draw artificial lines between the different parts and systems of the body. An honest inquiry into acupuncture can spur a paradigm shift and we stand on the threshold of that.[2]

---

1. Paradoxes in Acupuncture Research: Strategies for Moving Forward.
2. The Structure of Scientific Revolutions.

History

Not every art form stretches back to the beginning of recorded history quite like acupuncture does. Following the historical threads of acupuncture practice teaches us about their origins and how they were constructed. Tracking the flow upstream takes us back to the source.

> *"With regards to tracing upstream, only the Su Wen and the Nan Jing are the most important."*
> *Yang Jizhou, Essay on the Gains and Losses of the Various Schools, from the Zhenjiu Dacheng*

Learning the vast history of this medicine deepens it. Tracing it back to its roots and discerning the people, ideas, and events which shaped it is invigorating to our own modern practice of it. We stand on the shoulders of giants. Some left texts to convey their words, thoughts, and strategies to future generations. These were the generous acts of benevolent sages and those who wished to provide their knowledge to future generations.

Medicine is as old as humanity's mortality; ageless. From the beginning of time, death has followed humanity like its shadow. This art comes from the genuine desire of people to cure disease and prevent illness and death. Medicine is an existential balm on the soul of humanity. It is a tradition which has been broadened by numerous ages, cultures, peoples, and dynasties throughout time.

In some fields, there may be no reason to look back more than a handful of generations. Something unique about acupuncture is that it has evolved through thousands of years. It has weathered social, political, and ideological storms, survived, adapted, and grown. Yet after all these ages, one question remains: what will our generation add to this vast legacy?

Philosophy

Chinese medicine can fundamentally be understood as a practical application of classical Chinese philosophy. Rather than emerging as an isolated empirical science, it operationalized the abstract cosmological, metaphysical, and political theories of the late Zhou, Qin, and Han dynasties into a concrete, functioning system of human physiology, pathology, and therapy.

It is my belief that students of Chinese medicine should also study philosophy. Chinese philosophy forms the foundational substrate of many of the formative ideas of medicine; the logic, language, and values. Exposing the philosophical undercurrents injects vitality into our understanding; it broadens it and deepens it. The acupuncturist in many ways acts parallel to the philosophical sage by using the principles of Yin Yang, Wu Xing, and statecraft to restore order to the empire of the human body.

Not only will reading these great written works deepen our practice, but they may also deepen our personal lives in unforeseen ways. The philosophy books are also generally just a joy to read, and great works of literature in their own right. They are a deep source of wisdom; interesting and inspiring, they make us think about the world in new ways.

But this goes beyond Chinese philosophy alone, or any cultural school or system of knowledge, for that matter. In today's world, we have access to the greatest written works of all cultures and ages right at our fingertips! There has never been a better time to investigate the great ideas and wisdom traditions of human history, to learn, be curious, or to do comparative philosophy. So I would encourage anyone to take advantage of this opportunity in order to enrich our practice and our lives as a whole.

Confidence

"As is our confidence, so is our capacity."
William Hazlitt

As acupuncturists, we need to have confidence in the amazing ability of the human body to heal, and in acupuncture's abilities to stimulate a healing process reliably and effectively. We also have to have confidence in ourselves as practitioners. Confidence comes from continual practice, compounding experience, profound study, and experiencing repeated positive results. By genuinely striving to become proficient in our art, we build the confidence to meet most any situation. I believe that the work we do outside of the clinic, whether in study, thought, dialogue, or isolation, builds our confidence proportionally. Training and practicing are essential.

Although we may fail at times, and inevitably we will not always be successful, we must allow these lessons to be stepping stones which we humbly learn and become more competent from. In this sense, failure becomes a positive outcome because it builds our experience, provides us meaningful feedback, and develops us towards future successes. Competence breeds confidence, and "confidence can shape how we act and is optimized when it corresponds to reality".[1] Approach each new situation with healthy levels of humility, optimism, and confidence.

---

1. Confidence-competence alignment and the role of self-confidence in medical education: A conceptual review.

Humility

"The heavens are lasting and the earth is enduring. The reason the world is able to be lasting and enduring is because it does not live for itself. Thus it is able to be long-lived. It is on this model that the sages withdraw their persons from contention yet find themselves out in front. Put their own persons out of mind yet find themselves taken care of. Isn't it simply because they are unselfish that they can satisfy their own needs."
Dao De Jing, Chapter 7

As acupuncturists, we often step into a patient's life at moments of vulnerability—where pain, illness, or imbalance disrupt their sense of self and quality of life. We accompany individuals through the profound existential realities of being human: suffering, mortality, and the search for meaning. We are engaging with a person's Qi, and each one of us is a unique phenomenon which is finite and fleeting. Humility ensures one meets patients where they are, rather than where one assumes they should be. It fosters a reverence for the patient's journey.

"Whenever eminent physicians treat an illness, they must quiet the spirit and settle the will, they must be free of wants and desires, and they must first develop a heart full of great compassion and empathy. They must pledge themselves completely to relieving the suffering of all sentient beings."
Sun Si Miao

Humility allows us to recognize our own limits as we face the existential weight which comes along with medicine and the mortality of life. We cannot defy death, but we can intervene and enhance the quality of the time which our patients have. Humility prevents us from overpromising or clinging to outcomes, allowing us to focus on what truly matters: alleviating suffering, restoring dignity, and honoring their humanity.

> *"Shall I teach you what wisdom means? To know what you know and know what you do not know – that then is wisdom."*
> *Confucian Analects, Chapter 2.17*

Just like our patients, we are vulnerable to the same frailties and human imperfections. Humility can keep us grounded, with the understanding that we always have room to grow, learn, and change for the better. Humility is a route to increased knowledge and better decision making. It invites curiosity over dogma, compassion over judgment, and resilience over burnout. Humility counteracts the tendency to become prideful or egoistic in our practice. Simply put, is it not wise to be humble?

> *"A great defect in life is pride. The proud son is sure not to be filial, nor the proud minister loyal, nor the proud father affectionate, nor the proud friend faithful... one must not harbor any egoism in the mind. To do so means to have pride. The many good points about ancient sages are but selflessness. Being selfless, one is naturally humble. Humility is the foundation of all virtues, while pride is the chief of all vices."*
> *Wang Yangming*[1]

---

1. A Confucian Approach to Teaching Humility.

The Space

"Environments are not passive wrappings, but are, rather, active processes which are invisible."
Marshall McLuhan

Cultivating a true healing space is an important aspect of acupuncture which can be easily overlooked. Patients need to be able to find refuge in an environment separate from what is normal or habitual for them. Often, modern societal environments are toxic and contribute to the formation of their illness. The ability to remove oneself from 'normal' society's unconsciously negative environments by entering a healing space, which is a different medium with a different *culture* and energetic resonance, should not be underestimated. A change in energetic tone can be substantial and assist in initiating a process of relaxation and an openness to change.

Every aspect of a space can be mindfully and consciously curated by the practitioner for the central goal of facilitating a welcoming, safe, and healing environment for a patient. This can be an area where Feng Shui can be applied with great usefulness. Often, patients are used to medical environments which are intimidating, unwelcoming, cold, stifling, stagnant, or even oppressive on an unconscious level. The space can influence a patient's first impression and it can exert effects on the treatment experience itself. A warm and inviting space can increase the odds that a patient will want to continue with a habitual practice of acupuncture treatment. When we enter a genuinely healing space we can sense it.

Variables which can be considered are lighting, music, and scent, to name a few. We should be aware that some patients are extremely sensitive and that these *rarified* aspects of a space can be the difference between someone having a positive or negative experience. Choosing the objects and their placement in a space affects how it operates, because a space is a medium. Every medium creates different possibilities of creativity and exerts different constraints on what is possible in it. Just as a room which is pitch black will reduce the possibilities of what can be done with it, the many variables of a space will determine what is possible and can emerge from within it.[1]

A treatment space should reflect the goals of an acupuncture treatment. It should be a tranquil, safe place where people can relax and enter a state of quietude so that their spirits can be at peace. It should be a space where the practitioner can give their undivided attention to the patient, where observation, diagnosis, and treatment can be done without distractions. The space is carefully crafted to resonate with a state of harmony which imprints into anyone who enters it, synergizing with the ultimate goals of an acupuncture treatment.

---

1. Understanding Media: The Extensions of Man

Music

"Music washes away from the soul the dust of everyday life."
Berthold Auerbach

In ancient China, rites and music were the primary tools used by sage-kings to maintain social order, structure the political hierarchy, and morally transform the populace. Because music reflects the heart and the times, the health of a government could be diagnosed purely by listening to its music. Music possessed such raw power that it was believed to be physically dangerous if misused.

"As a general principle, music is the harmony between Heaven and Earth, and the perfect blend of Yin and Yang."
The Annals of Lü Buwei, Book 5 Chapter 2.3

Modern research independently confirms measurable physiological and psychological healing effects of music. For instance, music profoundly influences the default mode network, an important large-scale brain circuit. This is an attribute which directly overlaps with acupuncture, offering a potentially powerful synergy.

In general music acts as a mood regulator, fostering psycho-physical well-being and physical recovery. Slower tempo, simple melodies, and consonant intervals induce low arousal and positive feelings such as peacefulness and relaxation.[1] The right music sets the mood; it creates the environment; it lets people drop into an embodied experience. Music is a profound tool which we can utilize to cultivate and dial in the exact vibrational and energetic context we need for our work, and that we seek for our patients.

"Music has healing power. It has the ability to take people out of themselves for a few hours."
Elton John

Optimally, one should think of music not as a standalone cure, but as a powerful medium to assist in healing the whole person. It should be viewed as an integral part of a comprehensive, multi-disciplinary treatment and the healing experience, and it should certainly not be neglected when designing the ideal environment of a healing acupuncture treatment space.

---

1. Uncovering Potential Distinctive Acoustic Features of Healing Music

Listening

"Whoever has ears, let them hear.
Jesus, Matthew 13:9-16

Another way that we can pick up on the Image of the Qi is through listening to the subtle sounds and word choices which are on display by a patient. Not only should we be listening intently to what the patient is saying to us, but we should also be acutely aware of *how* it is being said. The tone of their voice, the emotive quality of their communications, and their choice of words, all betray the underlying operational patterns of Qi disharmony.

"The five depots appearing in the tones, they can be known by way of reasoning."
Su Wen, Chapter 10

Beyond diagnosis of systematic correspondences, listening is a core skill in the clinical encounter. Not everyone is a natural when it comes to listening and communication. "The ability to communicate effectively is not innate; it is a learned skill that requires ongoing practice and refinement."[1] Listening is something which we can practice and improve at.

One of the common complaints which patients have with the western medical experience is that they feel like doctors don't listen to them. One study found that doctors interrupt patients every eleven seconds.[2] The takeaway for me is that there is often a lot of value and benefit to listening more and talking less. I think this applies generally to life as well.

> *"Deep listening is the kind of listening that can help relieve the suffering of another person. You can call it compassionate listening. You listen only with one purpose: to help him or her empty their heart... because you know by listening like that, you give that person a chance to suffer less."*
> *Thich Nhat Hanh*

When a patient tells me something or tries to express something to me, it is often very meaningful. I am not saying to mindlessly do whatever a patient says; on the contrary, I am advocating for teamwork and collaboration. It is not uncommon that a patient will tell me what they need, sometimes even unconsciously. Tuning in to these transmissions can create a better experience and outcomes for them. Patients will feel heard, we will build better rapport, and we may intuit treatment paths which we would not have thought of otherwise.

---

1. Active Listening
2. Eliciting the Patient's Agenda- Secondary Analysis of Recorded Clinical Encounters

Scent

The sense of smell is an important diagnostic tool which is often overlooked, though it was prized and valued in the classics. Disharmonies and disorders, manifesting themselves holistically, will present outwardly in ways distinguishable by all of the senses. The scent which is given off by a patient is a clue to their inner bodily ecology, and it is a microcosmic sign of their holographic pattern of disharmony. This scent can be subtle or overt, depending upon the severity of the case. Sensitive practitioners should be on the alert for these important clues, which can give compelling diagnostic insights into the Image of Qi that is operating and underlying their disorder. There are times when the scent of a patient immediately alerts me to an underlying disharmony. Sometimes, picking up on a scent can be the keystone to making a diagnosis which is otherwise complex and opaque.

> *The Heart masters odors. Entering itself, it manifests a scorched odor. Entering the Spleen, it manifests a fragrant odor. Entering the Liver, it manifests a rancid odor. Entering the Kidney, it manifests a putrid odor. Entering the Lung, it manifests a fishy odor.*
> *Zhenjiu Dacheng*

Feeling and Palpation

"From feeling one can obtain a hold. Inspect the vessel ruling the disease. When it is firm and has blood, and when it has sunk down, in both cases one gets a hold of the disease by feeling the vessel."
Su Wen, Chapter 39

The sense of touch is one of the most powerful tools we have at our disposal for diagnostics. Feeling the pulse, with all of its subtle nuances, is the quintessential part of this procedure. Engendering and developing sensitivity in the fingertips and being able to correlate the pulse to inner states of Qi turns the hands of the acupuncturist into a potent organic Qi imaging device.

However, palpation goes beyond even taking the pulse. Using our hands to feel the channels and the tissues can help guide our understanding of the nature of an illness or injury. We need to be able to distinguish between tissues, find nuanced locations, and diagnose healthy and sick areas, all with our hands. It can help us to locate and identify the most active, living points for treatment; locations of excess or deficiency, vacuity or conglomeration.

Let's not forget that feeling and sensitivity are equally important during the act of needling itself. We must be aware of the arrival of the Qi. Our sense of touch must extend through the needle itself and beyond, through to the body of the patient. When the Qi arrives, the needle will feel differently than when it does not. Developing a sensitivity of feeling is essential and comes with experience; the more patients we see and pulses we palpate, the faster it will develop.

"When the Qì has already arrived, then the needle becomes rough and tight, resembling a fish swallowing a baited hook, with a sinking or floating

movement; if their Qì does not come, the needle is surely light or smooth, and it is like residing inside of a still, unoccupied room, silent, where nothing can be heard."

The Ode of Mysterious Indications, from the Zhenjiu Dacheng

Healing Touch

Beyond using touch as palpation for diagnostic purposes, acupuncturists should not forget that touch itself has healing benefits and properties.[1] There is something ancient and primordial about the healing nature of touch — we all know how good it feels to have attention given to our pains in the form of touch. Acupressure and massage are themselves important components of Chinese medicine. The healing aspects of touch can imbue even the diagnostic portion of an acupuncture session with healing elements. During the process of palpating channels and acupuncture points, and identifying active areas of treatment, we are provided with a prime opportunity to apply healing touch to those areas.

A patient's body may have been deprived of a healing, caring touch for a lengthy amount of time. In many cases, patients often neglect and ignore their own bodies. Teaching them to apply simple aspects of healing touch, such as acupressure or simple massage techniques, on important points or channels, gives them the opportunity to apply healing touch on their own. This can bring agency back to a patient who may not have a concept of how to go about their own self-care. It can also open their horizons to new ways of healing themselves through self-massage or acupressure, and develop the connection they have to their body and its pain.

The concept of healing touch is an ancient one which harkens back to ideas such as the 'laying on of hands', though healing touch does not need to have those religious connotations, and it is not contingent upon the beliefs of the patient. Touch can stimulate psycho-neuro-endocrine modulation in a patient's entire system.[2] The idea of engaging with the patient's bio-energetic and physical body through touch is a powerful one which grounds our practice in our hands. Touch has long been part of the traditional methods of acupuncture practice: grasping, pressing, rubbing, massaging, guiding and stroking along the channels. Finding ways to integrate even simple aspects of healing touch into our treatment process opens up an important new dimension to our practice.

"If the painful spot has not yet been eliminated, promptly stroke and rub the painful spot to make the pain scatter."
Zhenjiu Dacheng

---

1. Therapeutic touch: a healing modality.
2. The Neurophysiological Impact of Touch-Based Therapy: Insights and Clinical Benefits.

Emotions

Emotions are a very insubstantial but powerful form of Qi. Emotions color the human experience and even animate the body, but they are also one of the primary causes of disease. The powerful effect which they exert on the whole system can send it to extremes. When emotions are intense, the Qi responds accordingly.

> *"I know that the hundred diseases are generated by the Qi. When one is angry, then the Qi rises. When one is joyous, then the Qi relaxes. When one is sad, then the Qi dissipates. When one is in fear, then the Qi moves down. In case of cold the Qi collects. In case of heat the Qi flows out. When one is frightened, then the Qi is in disorder. When one is exhausted, then the Qi is wasted. When one is pensive, then the Qi lumps together."*
> *Su Wen, Chapter 39*

Both the absence of emotion as well as the overwhelming of emotion are neither ideal nor sustainable states of being, regardless of which emotion we are referring to. This is why the sages were calm and tranquil. One of the reasons why they lived so long is because their emotional state was not disordered, and so they were in a harmonious state of being.

> *"Sages are like a mirror — they neither see things off nor go out to meet them, they respond to everything without storing anything up. They are thus never injured through the myriad transformations they undergo."*
> *Zhuangzi, Chapter 7*

Emotions are a natural part of life but ideally they must come and go at appropriate times and at appropriate levels. Being flooded with emotion for extended periods of time is not sustainable. Being completely devoid of emotion makes life empty and gray. Emotional regulation is essential to health and longevity. Excessive emotional indulgence directly causes disease.

> *"The fact is, grief, anxiety, overthinking and worry injure the Heart.... anger and rage counterflow Qì upwards and not downwards, injuring the Liver."*
> *Commentary on the Nan Jing, from the Zhenjiu Dacheng*

Acupuncture has the ability to regulate and harmonize the Qi and thus it exerts its effects even on such subtle and diaphanous phenomena as the emotions. An example of this can be seen in the effects acupuncture has on the brain and the nervous system. Acupuncture can modulate the limbic system and other interrelated neural networks. "These limbic structures are central to the regulation and control of emotion, cognition, bio-behavior, endocrine and autonomic nervous functions, and are activated by stress, pain and emotions of negative valence."[1] Dysregulation of these systems is implicated in major depression and mood disorders when hyperreactive. This means that acupuncture could play a profound role in a large subset of mood-related disorders.

---

1. Acupuncture, the Limbic System, and the Anticorrelated Networks of the Brain

Vision

To see the patient is to know them. Visual acuity and perception are cornerstones to diagnosis. The art of visual observation is mentioned repeatedly in the classics.

> "Someone who looks at the [patient's] complexion and knows his disease, he is called enlightened."[1]
> *Ling Shu, Chapter 4*

Through their complexion and tissues, subtle colors shimmer and emanate as notes of disharmony. This resonance unveils their state to a keen, discerning eye. This is a function of resonance and interconnectedness; disharmonies in physiological systems can present themselves through the various colors or visual abnormalities. We should be very discerning in our vision, and observe their complexions with keen eyes, in order to notice important diagnostic information.

> *"Complexion and flavors match the five depots. White matches the lung and acrid. Red matches the heart and bitter. Green-blue matches the liver and sour. Yellow matches the spleen and sweet. Black matches the kidneys and salty."*
> *Su Wen, Chapter 10*

Images of Qi manifest themselves through various means observable by the senses. When we see these images, we gain insight into the deeper nature of the situation and its propensities. Visual signs can be clues pointing to deeper anomalies such as organ-system disharmonies.

> *"The phenomena associated with the conditions of the five depots, they can be deduced from objects of the same kind."*
> *Su Wen, Chapter 10*

Red flares of inflammation, pale shadows of deficiency, or dark pools of stagnation—these resonant Qi images emerge for us to read. Vision is one of the most important tools in our diagnostic repertoire to study and practice. Combining vision with pulse, sound, scent, and touch, we can begin to corroborate patterns and paint a coherent image of Qi.

> *"Those who are able to match the movement in the vessels and the complexion, they can achieve success in a myriad of cases."*
> *Su Wen, Chapter 10*

We may tend to prioritize vision over the other senses, but I think it is important to remember that it is just one of the many senses at our disposal. In fact, we might think of the tradition of blind acupuncturists, long revered in Japan. Each of us may have certain senses which are the most naturally acutely sensitive. For some, perhaps that is vision; for others, it could be sound, touch, or scent. Each of us can find our own strengths and we can develop them and rely upon them in the clinic.

---

1. See also Nan Jing, Chapter 61.

Intuition

Strive to bring intuition into the practice. Intuition is essential for any creative art form, and acupuncture is no exception. Be on the lookout for cues from the universe, hidden synchronicities, random sparks of insight and ideas.

The ability to follow intuition is essential to go with the flow, to follow the principle of Wu Wei or 'non-doing'. To be rigid in how we do things, inflexible or stuck in a routine and structure, or trapped by a fixed method or plan, is not ideal. To resist intuition and the creative flow of ideas is to miss important opportunities which present themselves. Intuition brings a softness and a Yin nature.

> *"What is too hard snaps, and what is too soft folds: the Way is right between hardness and softness."*
> *Wen Zi, Chapter 153*

Something a patient says can inspire an idea for a point to use. They may even intuit a point somewhere would be beneficial themselves. If there is no reason to say no, why not say yes? Allow synchronicities to manifest. These may be important intuitions which are flowing naturally between patient and practitioner during the healing encounter. Entertain the unorthodox creative possibilities they bring.

Be flexible enough to incorporate the unexpected into one's plans or methods. Getting stuck in a pattern of treatment breeds stiffness and rigidity. It actually feels good to break out of a fixed pattern, like a breath of fresh air. Prescriptions and protocols are useful, but a formula which never alters or transforms to the situation becomes brittle and one dimensional over time. Cultivating openness to intuition allows for new light to enter into whatever we do.

Authenticity

Strive to be authentic. Authenticity is an essential trait which patients appreciate, even subconsciously. Who wants to get acupuncture from someone who is not genuinely passionate about it? Who feels like they aren't being real with us? Acupuncture needs to be an integral part of your life, beyond mere curiosity, bordering on an obsession. Whatever we do in life, obsession is mandatory. If it is something you find authentically interesting, cool, and fun, then this will be felt by others naturally. If it is not an authentic passion, something which we live and breathe, both in and out of the clinic, then people will feel that.

> *"But to express oneself honestly, not lying to oneself...now that, my friend, is very hard to do."*
> *Bruce Lee*

Compassion

Compassion is a necessary component to being a health care practitioner, and it pulls us in a direction towards becoming better acupuncturists. The benevolent feeling we have towards our patients will compel us to do our utmost for them. As human beings we are all flawed and imperfect, mortal beings. Meeting people with a sense of compassion is humane and appropriate when confronting illness, pain, and disease.

Patients are actively looking for a sense of compassion from their healthcare practitioners. It is one of the biggest criticisms of modern healthcare that it feels cold and lacking in compassion.[1] Being able to provide compassionate care is an important part of the relationship we build with patients. If they do not feel as though we genuinely care for them, then how can we expect them to build a relationship of mutual trust and respect with us? How can we expect them to be vulnerable and share necessary details of their history, or to be forthcoming with us? Or follow our recommendations and treatment guidelines? Compassion and empathy create a foundation for rapport.

> *"I have three treasures to hold and to keep: The first is compassion."*
> *Dao De Jing Chapter 67*

---

1. Compassion: A Scoping Review of the Healthcare Literature.

Do No Harm

"Practice two things in your dealings with disease: either help or do not harm the patient."
Hippocrates, Epidemics, Book I

By some estimates, iatrogenesis, which is the unintentional cause of injury or illness by a medical practitioner, is the fifth leading cause of death worldwide.[1] But the idea that medicine and doctors can be a source of harm is not a new idea. The Classics often speak about the importance of correct practice in order to avoid injury to patients. Despite acupuncture being a profoundly safe practice in the modern age, this is still an ethical lesson which we must fully bear in our hearts on a daily basis.

If a practitioner fails to understand the "end and beginning" of the channels (the boundaries of entry and exit), they will inevitably treat repletion as depletion or mistake evil Qi for true Qi. This clinical error acts as a "Qi bandit"—it drains the patient's remaining true Qi and leaves the pathogenic evil to take exclusive, permanent possession of the interior, cutting short the patient's life.
The Systematic Classic of Acupuncture and Moxibustion

Given that medical error is one of the leading causes of death, acupuncturists have the profound opportunity to provide a healing service which runs counter to this trend. In our practice, we can strive for safety and excellence, executing skillful treatments with sincerity. We even have our own models of ethical leadership in figures such as Sun Simiao, who developed ethical precepts during the Tang Dynasty which still remain relevant today.[2]

(1) A physician's duty is to heal the wounded and rescue the dying, and to relieve their sufferings. No matter how rich and how poor they are, patients are treated equally.

(2) Never be afraid of difficulties and danger and wholeheartedly strive to rescue patients.

(3) Never be disgusted by filth and stench in the treatment of patients.

(4) Give careful and accurate diagnosis, keep calm, and pay attention to the patient's safety.

(5) Show great respect for peers and never be jealous of others.

By practicing the profound lessons of our healing art, mastering the methods and techniques of diagnosis and treatment, and studying the wisdom and ethical guidance of the masters and sages, we endeavor to behave righteously as leaders with the well being of our patients always at the center of our actions.

> *"When the Qi move contrary to the norms and when the disease increases in severity in the course of repeated piercings, that has nothing to do with Yin and Yang Qi, or their potential at the surface and in the depth. These are always destructions caused by unrefined [healers], i.e., misdeeds of a practitioner."*
> *Ling Shu, Chapter 67*

---

1. Iatrogenesis: A review on nature, extent, and distribution of healthcare hazards

2. Sun Simiao, Super Physician of the Tang Dynasty

Having Fun

"I know of no other way of associating with great tasks than play: as a sign of greatness, this is an essential presupposition."
Nietzsche

Can we say that we are truly successful if we are not enjoying ourselves? Having fun is important for the health and the sustainability of any practice. It is also integral for how effective that practice is, and how long it can be sustained without burning out.

It is fun when we can figure out how to make things work, when our methods are effective. When we can be creative, and when our work is akin to play. Let us remember the initial feeling of curiosity and wonder which sent us down our path. We should be having fun with our art, even though at times it can be challenging, and even when there are obstacles. Have fun overcoming the obstacles. The way we frame our perspective towards it can determine a lot about how we experience it. Let the joy of the work sink in.

Treat practice as though it were play. Enjoy practice; get comfortable in it and savor the experience of growth and development. It is the process of becoming. There can be a depth to play when it is playfulness towards an important goal or trajectory. "The deep plays are those which are moved by the heights."[1] Learning new ways of doing things, finding new solutions to problems, using creativity to experiment and innovate: when people's problems start going away, it is very fun, and they are very happy.

Another thing to think about as well is that our patients should also be having a fun, enjoyable experience. While it is true that acupuncture can cause some feeling of discomfort and we are often dealing with pain itself, the overall experience should be such that the patient actually wants to return. Acupuncture should be something they actively look forward to practicing again. Part of this occurs naturally, as our enthusiasm rubs off on them infectiously, or they see their issues resolve. But if we step into our patient's shoes, we might remember the novelty and curiosity of our own first acupuncture experience. We are bringing them into a different world, exposing them to new knowledge and ways of thinking or being, and giving them insights into their problems. The act of acupuncture can be made fun as we explain the important elements, shine a light on what is happening, and unveil some of the mystery of their body and their situation to them. Many patients are extremely curious about acupuncture, and they relish the chance to glean insights and knowledge about themselves and their acupuncture experience. I like to bring a little bit of humor, playfulness, and humanity into the treatment experience.

Medicine is serious business. Health, illness, and mortality, are obviously grave issues of importance. If we can enjoy the process of learning, practicing medicine, and performing acupuncture, it will be sustainable and give us sustenance. Those who enjoy their work are truly blessed. Acupuncture practice and self-cultivation are a life-long process, and having fun with it will produce the best and longest lasting results.

---

1. You Must Change Your Life.

Experimentation

"We are experiments: let us also want to be such!"
Nietzsche

We have to be willing to try new things. Not everything is going to always work, and that is okay, as long as we are trying our best. Sometimes, trying our best requires us to experiment with new ideas, new techniques, new concepts, or new approaches. This is how we find new ways to fix problems. Trying new things and experimenting is part of practicing any art. We have to be willing to fail sometimes, if we are going to find out the ways to succeed consistently. Experimentation is an essential part of the creative process. The proclivity for creativity and experimentation is often tied to the openness to experience personality trait, and research shows that openness predicts creative achievement in the arts, distinct from the trait that predicts achievement in the sciences. If we treat acupuncture as the art form it is, cultivating this openness isn't incidental to our practice, it's foundational to it.[1] A practice which does not make room for experimentation remains stale, and growth is slow. Look for opportunities to try new things, especially when we encounter problems where we don't have the perfect solution or method. Life itself can be treated experimentally.

---

1. Openness to Experience and Intellect Differentially Predict Creative Achievement in the Arts and Sciences.

Patient Centeredness

At the center of the entire equation and overall goal of medicine is the patient. The purpose of medicine is to improve the quality of life of the patient by alleviating their disease, or pain, or whatever is disrupting the harmony of their life. It is easy for this simple fact to become occluded in the modern day, where medicine is ensconced within economics, politics, ideology, personal ambition, desires, and numerous other drives and motivations.

Listening to our patients attentively, communicating with them in ways which create genuine understanding and learning, and creating real space for them to ask meaningful questions, invites them to become active participants and collaborators in the acupuncture experience we are facilitating for them. The patient and the practitioner ideally work together as a team. We can learn to tailor our communications to different patients in ways which meet each of them where they are at, rather than expect them to enter into our highly technical and specialist culture, which can be complex and is often very foreign to them. When working with patients, we should inquire into and respect their preferences, as well as take an active interest in them and their particular needs.

The center of any clinical enterprise must always be the patients themselves.[1] Beyond just the acupuncture, the entire clinical enterprise can be tailored to this center. This involves basic operations such as scheduling, payment, and customer service, to the layout and design of the physical space itself. Every detail can be tailored to optimize the experience of the patient by placing them at the center and asking ourselves, 'what would create the best experience for our patients?'

---

1. Crossing the Quality Chasm: A New Health System for the 21st Century.

Mortality

"Medicine is the arbiter of human life, none but those with high ideals and moral integrity should practice it. The principles of acupuncture are profound and subtle, one must depend upon the teachings and guidance of fully realized human sages."
The Ode to the Hundred Disorders, from the Zhenjiu Dacheng

Life is finite, and death is inevitable. It is a natural phase in the endless cycle of the cosmos, the dispersion of our Qi, the exhaustion of our Jing, and thus the end of our individual potential. Our work entails nourishing life, assisting life, regulating life, but also acknowledging the finality and ultimate mortality which awaits us all. The patients we treat, the people who we form relationships with, as well as ourselves, will all die. There is nothing we can do to stop it; this is the natural course of life. Medicine is about nourishing the full allotment of life, assisting to manifest the individual's utmost potential, and their ability to age gracefully.

"When you don't yet understand life, how can you understand death?"
Confucius

Our job may be to prolong life and encourage the benefits of a long existence, to avert premature death and disaster, and to increase the quality of life through the reduction of pain and the minimizing of sickness, but we should also contemplate death and mortality and practice facing it with equanimity. By contemplating death, we may better appreciate and utilize the finite time we have with gratitude and humility, and make every moment we experience more poignant and meaningful.

> *"The Great Clod burdens me with form, labors me with life, eases me in old age, and rests me in death."*
> *Zhuangzi*

Mortality and aging represent the gradual loss of an organism's ability to maintain its complex, out-of-equilibrium organization. It is finally complete when the system's boundaries and internal closure of constraints break down. Death occurs when the body's internal bureaucracy collapses. All empires eventually fall. No longer able to resist the universal pull of entropy, the biological system inevitably attains complete equilibrium. In a sense, we can think of death as the ultimate state of balance. The Spirit fully departs, the physical form is rendered an inert shell, and the process of life and death is complete.

References

Ader, R. Psychoneuroimmunology. 4th Edition. Academic Press. October 10, 2011.

Abuhamdeh S. Investigating the "Flow" Experience: Key Conceptual and Operational Issues. Front Psychol. 2020 Feb 13;11:158. doi: 10.3389/fpsyg.2020.00158. PMID: 32116954; PMCID: PMC7033418.

Ames, R., Hall, D. Dao De Jing: A Philosophical Translation (English and Mandarin Chinese Edition). Ballantine Books; English and Mandarin Chinese Edition, December 30, 2003.

Ames, R., Rosemont, H. The Analects of Confucius: A Philosophical Translation (Classics of Ancient China). Ballantine Books; 1st edition, September 7, 1999.

Andrew, A., LaFleur, R.A. Remonstrance: The Moral Imperative of the Chinese Scholar-Official. The Association for Asian Studies. Volume 19:2 (Fall 2014): Maritime Asia. Accessed July 3, 2026. https://www.asianstudies.org/publications/eaa/archives/remonstrance-the-moral-imperative-of-the-chinese-scholar-official/

Auerbach, Berthold. *On the Heights*. Translated by Fanny Elizabeth Bunnett. New York: Leypoldt & Holt, 1867.

Bensky, D., Scheid, V., Ellis, A., Barolet, R. Chinese Herbal Medicine Formulas and Strategies, 2nd Ed. Eastland Press, 2009.

Bonanno M, Papa GA, Calabrò RS. The Neurophysiological Impact of Touch-Based Therapy: Insights and Clinical Benefits. J Integr Neurosci. 2024 Dec 11;23(12):214. doi: 10.31083/j.jin2312214. PMID: 39735966.

Browne, William (1590–1645). "Variety."

Calvino, Italo. "Why Read the Classics?" In *Why Read the Classics?*, translated by Martin McLaughlin, 3–9. New York: Pantheon Books, 1999.

Chan, W. A Source Book in Chinese Philosophy. Princeton University Press. April 1, 1969.

Christoffersen VR, Škodlar B, Henriksen MG. Exploring tranquility: Eastern and Western perspectives. Front Psychol. 2022 Aug 1;13:931827. doi: 10.3389/fpsyg.2022.931827. PMID: 35978784; PMCID: PMC9376312.

Cleary, T. The Book of Balance and Harmony. Shambhala, November 11, 2003.

Cleary, T. Wen-Tzu: Understanding the Mysteries. Shambhala; Reprint edition, September 29, 1992.

Covey, Stephen R. *The 7 Habits of Highly Effective People: Powerful Lessons in Personal Change*. New York: Simon and Schuster, 1989.

Csikszentmihalyi, M. Flow: The Psychology of Optimal Experience. Harper Perennial Modern Classics; 1st edition. July 1, 2008.

De Bary, W.T., Bloom, I., Adler, J. Sources of Chinese Tradition, Vol. 1: From Earliest times to 1600. Columbia University Press. July 1, 1999.

De Bary, W.T., Lufrano, R. Sources of Chinese Tradition, Vol. 2: From 1600 Through the Twentieth Century. Columbia University Press. January 1, 1999.

Deadman, P. et al. Manual of Acupuncture. Journal of Chinese Medicine Publications, 2007. 2nd Edition.

Deleuze, Gilles, and Félix Guattari. *A Thousand Plateaus: Capitalism and Schizophrenia*. Translated by Brian Massumi. Minneapolis: University of Minnesota Press, 1987.

Denmei, Shudō. Finding Effective Acupuncture Points. Eastland Pr; 1st edition. February 3, 2003.

Descartes, René. *Discourse on the Method*. In *The Philosophical Writings of Descartes, Volume 1*, translated by John Cottingham, Robert Stoothoff, and Dugald Murdoch, 111–151. Cambridge: Cambridge University Press, 1985.

Dharmananda, S. Bleeding Peripheral Points: An Acupuncture Technique. ITM Online. Accessed March 24, 2025. http://www.itmonline.org/arts/bleeding.htm

Ding Y, Jing J, Guo Q, Zhou J, Cheng X, Chen X, Wang L, Tang Y, Fan Q. Uncovering potential distinctive acoustic features of healing music. Gen Psychiatr. 2023 Nov 7;36(6):e101145. doi: 10.1136/gpsych-2023-101145. PMID: 38155842; PMCID: PMC10753712.

Dong-Yuan, L. Treatise on the Spleen and Stomach: A Translation of the Pi Wei Lun. Blue Poppy Press. January 1, 1993.

Doucet BM, Lam A, Griffin L. Neuromuscular electrical stimulation for skeletal muscle function. Yale J Biol Med. 2012 Jun;85(2):201-15. Epub 2012 Jun 25. PMID: 22737049; PMCID: PMC3375668.

Durant, Will. *The Story of Philosophy: The Lives and Opinions of the Greater Philosophers*. New York: Simon and Schuster, 1926.

Durrant, Stephen, Wai-yee Li, and David Schaberg, trans. and eds. The Zuo Tradition / Zuozhuan Reader: Selections from China's Earliest Narrative History. Seattle: University of Washington Press, 2020.

Feynman, Richard P. *The Character of Physical Law*. MIT Press, 1965.

Gleick, James, and Eliot Porter. *Nature's Chaos*. Viking, 1990.

Gottlieb M, Chan TM, Zaver F, Ellaway R. Confidence-competence alignment and the role of self-confidence in medical education: A conceptual review. Med Educ. 2022 Jan;56(1):37-47. doi: 10.1111/medu.14592. Epub 2021 Jul 20. PMID: 34176144.

Han J. S. (2004). Acupuncture and endorphins. Neuroscience letters, 361(1-3), 258–261. https://doi.org/10.1016/j.neulet.2003.12.019

Hazlitt, William. *Characteristics: In the Manner of Rochefoucault's Maxims*. London: John Templeman, 1837.

Hippocrates. *Epidemics I and III*. Translated by W. H. S. Jones. Loeb Classical Library. Cambridge, MA: Harvard University Press, 1923.

Ho, Mae-Wan. "Coherent Energy, Liquid Crystallinity and Acupuncture." Talk presented to the British Acupuncture Society, October 2, 1999. Institute of Science in Society, i-sis.org.uk.

Hui KK, Marina O, Liu J, Rosen BR, Kwong KK. Acupuncture, the limbic system, and the anticorrelated networks of the brain. Auton Neurosci. 2010 Oct 28;157(1-2):81-90. doi: 10.1016/j.autneu.2010.03.022. Epub 2010 May 21. PMID: 20494627; PMCID: PMC3754836.

Institute of Medicine. *Crossing the Quality Chasm: A New Health System for the 21st Century*. Washington, DC: National Academies Press, 2001.

Jing-Nuan, W. Ling Shu or The Spiritual Pivot. Univ of Hawaii Pr; Enlarged edition. January 1, 2002.

John, Elton. Interview by Jake Shears. "When Elton Met Jake." *The Guardian*, August 21, 2006.

Kaufman, Scott Barry, et al. "Openness to Experience and Intellect Differentially Predict Creative Achievement in the Arts and Sciences." *Journal of Personality* 84, no. 2 (2016): 248–258.

Keane, M. Covid: A Modern Form of Gu Syndrome: A Chinese Herbal Medicine Theory Handbook. Michael Keane Creative Studios. March 5, 2024.

Keane, M. Zhen Jiu Da Cheng. As of yet unpublished translations - future release pending publication by Michael Keane Creative Studios.

Kim, J. Zhang Zai's Philosophy of Qi: A Practical Understanding. Lexington Books. March 6, 2015.

Knoblock, J., Riegel, J. The Annals of Lü Buwei. Stanford University Press; 1st edition, January 1, 2001.

Konieczny L, Roterman-Konieczna I, Spólnik P. Systems Biology: Functional Strategies of Living Organisms [Internet]. 2nd edition. Cham (CH): Springer; 2023. Chapter 1, The Structure and Function of Living Organisms. 2023 Jun 9. Available from: https://www.ncbi.nlm.nih.gov/books/NBK599595/ doi: 10.1007/978-3-031-31557-2_1

Kreitzer MJ, Gross CR, Waleekhachonloet OA, Reilly-Spong M, Byrd M. The brief serenity scale: a psychometric analysis of a measure of spirituality and well-being. J Holist Nurs. 2009 Mar;27(1):7-16. doi: 10.1177/0898010108327212. Epub 2009 Jan 28. PMID: 19176898; PMCID: PMC2818779.

Kuhn, T. The Structure of Scientific Revolutions: 50th Anniversary Edition. University of Chicago Press; Fourth edition. April 30, 2012.

Lam, C. M. (2023). A Confucian approach to teaching humility. *Educational Philosophy and Theory*, *55*(2), 207–216. https://doi.org/10.1080/00131857.2022.2112032

Langevin HM, Churchill DL, Cipolla MJ. Mechanical signaling through connective tissue: a mechanism for the therapeutic effect of acupuncture. FASEB J. 2001 Oct;15(12):2275-82. doi: 10.1096/fj.01-0015hyp. PMID: 11641255.

Langevin HM, Wayne PM, Macpherson H, Schnyer R, Milley RM, Napadow V, Lao L, Park J, Harris RE, Cohen M, Sherman KJ, Haramati A, Hammerschlag R. Paradoxes in acupuncture research: strategies for moving forward. Evid Based Complement Alternat Med. 2011;2011:180805. doi: 10.1155/2011/180805. Epub 2010 Oct 11. PMID: 20976074; PMCID: PMC2957136.

Li M, Liang Y, Sun Simiao, Super Physician of the Tang Dynasty, Journal of Traditional Chinese Medical Sciences (2016), http://dx.doi.org/10.1016/j.jtcms.2016.01.005.

Lin YJ, Kung YY, Kuo WJ, Niddam DM, Chou CC, Cheng CM, Yeh TC, Hsieh JC, Chiu JH. Effect of acupuncture 'dose' on modulation of the default mode network of the brain. Acupunct Med. 2016 Dec;34(6):425-432. doi: 10.1136/acupmed-2016-011071. Epub 2016 Oct 6. PMID: 27841974; PMCID: PMC5256125.

Liu S, Bai Y, Liu J, Chen X, Lv P, Wang Y, Wang D and Wang S (2026) Decoding the mechanisms of acupuncture by neuroimaging: an integrated review from networks to molecules. Front. Hum. Neurosci. 20:1704570. doi: 10.3389/fnhum.2026.1704570.

Liu Yiming. *Cantong Qi Jing Wen Zhi Zhi* [Direct Pointing at the Scripture Text of the *Cantong Qi*]. 1799. Chinese Text Project, ctext.org/wiki.pl?if=en&chapter=108580.

López D, Vlamakis H, Kolter R. Biofilms. Cold Spring Harb Perspect Biol. 2010 Jul;2(7):a000398. doi: 10.1101/cshperspect.a000398. Epub 2010 Jun 2. PMID: 20519345; PMCID: PMC2890205.

MacPherson H, Vertosick EA, Foster NE, Lewith G, Linde K, Sherman KJ, Witt CM, Vickers AJ; Acupuncture Trialists' Collaboration. The persistence of the effects of acupuncture after a course of treatment: a meta-analysis of patients with chronic pain. Pain. 2017 May;158(5):784-793. doi: 10.1097/j.pain.0000000000000747. PMID: 27764035; PMCID: PMC5393924.

Maher, J.H. Advanced Tung Style Acupuncture: The Dao Ma Needling Technique of Master Tung Ching-Chang. RBC, January 1, 2005.

Major, J.S., et al. The Huainanzi: A Guide to the Theory and Practice of Government in Early Han China. Columbia University Press. April 14, 2010.

Matsumoto, K. & Birch, S. Extraordinary Vessels. Paradigm Publications. November 1, 1993.

McCann, H. Pricking the Vessels: Bloodletting Therapy in Chinese Medicine. Jessica Kingsley Publishers; Illustrated edition, February 28, 2014.

McLuhan, M. Understanding Media: The Extensions of Man. Signet Books; 2nd Edition, January 1, 1964.

Merton, T. The Way of Chuang Tzu. New Directions, 1965.

Messori, C. (2019) Deep into the Water: Exploring the Hydro-Electromagnetic and Quantum Electrodynamic Properties of Interfacial Water in Living Systems. Open Access Library Journal, 6: e5435. https://doi.org/10.4236/oalib.1105435

Merriam-Webster Dictionary. *Syncretism*. Accessed December 27, 2024. https://www.merriam-webster.com/dictionary/syncretism.

Mitchell, S. Tao Te Ching: A New English Version. Harper Perennial; Compact edition, January 1, 1988.

Montévil M, Mossio M. Biological organisation as closure of constraints. J Theor Biol. 2015 May 7;372:179-91. doi: 10.1016/j.jtbi.2015.02.029. Epub 2015 Mar 6. PMID: 25752259.

Mulloney, S. S., & Wells-Federman, C. (1996). Therapeutic touch: A healing modality. *Journal of Cardiovascular Nursing, 10*(3), 27–49.

Nhat Hanh, Thich. *True Love: A Practice for Awakening the Heart*. Boston: Shambhala Publications, 1997.

Nietzsche, Friedrich. *Daybreak: Thoughts on the Prejudices of Morality*. Translated by R. J. Hollingdale. Cambridge: Cambridge University Press, 1982.

Nietzsche, Friedrich. *Ecce Homo: How One Becomes What One Is*. Translated by Walter Kaufmann. In *On the Genealogy of Morals and Ecce Homo*. New York: Vintage Books, 1967.

Ovid. *Ars Amatoria* (*The Art of Love*), Book II, line 345.

Panda SK, da Silva LCN. Editorial: Understanding biofilms: recent trends and developments. Front Cell Infect Microbiol. 2025 Feb 11;15:1566230. doi: 10.3389/fcimb.2025.1566230. PMID: 40007611; PMCID: PMC11850994.

Park JE, Ryu YH, Liu Y, Jung HJ, Kim AR, Jung SY, Choi SM. A literature review of de qi in clinical studies. Acupunct Med. 2013 Jun;31(2):132-42. doi: 10.1136/acupmed-2012-010279. Epub 2013 Mar 13. PMID: 23486017; PMCID: PMC3686265.

Peer, R. F., & Shabir, N. (2018). Iatrogenesis: A review on nature, extent, and distribution of healthcare hazards. Journal of family medicine and primary care, 7(2), 309–314. https://doi.org/10.4103/jfmpc.jfmpc_329_17.

Prigogine, Ilya, and Isabelle Stengers. *Order Out of Chaos: Man's New Dialogue with Nature*. Bantam Books, 1984.

Ren, Y. B., Huang, J. H., Cai, W. J., & Shen, Z. Y. (2019). Shen-Jing as a Chinese Medicine Concept Might Be a Counterpart of Stem Cells in Regenerative Medicine. Chinese journal of integrative medicine, 25(1), 64–70. https://doi.org/10.1007/s11655-015-2136-z

Rickett, A.W. Guanzi: Political, Economic, and Philosophical Essays from Early China (Princeton Library of Asian Translations). Princeton University Press (August 31, 2021)

Rochat de la Vallée, Élisabeth. A Vision of the Origin of Qi Through Wind and Flavours. Journal of Chinese Medicine. JCM 115-13. Accessed March 21, 2025.

Schrödinger, E. What is Life? Cambridge University Press; Reprint edition, March 26, 2012.

Selye, Hans. *The Stress of Life*. McGraw-Hill, 1956.

Sennett, Richard. *The Craftsman*. New Haven: Yale University Press, 2008.

Sima Qian. Records of the Grand Historian: Qin Dynasty. Translated by Burton Watson. New York: Columbia University Press, 1993.

Sinclair, Shane, Jill M. Norris, Shelagh J. McConnell, Harvey Max Chochinov, Thomas F. Hack, Neil A. Hagen, Susan McClement, and Shelley Raffin Bouchal. "Compassion: A Scoping Review of the Healthcare Literature." *BMC Palliative Care* 15 (2016): 6. https://doi.org/10.1186/s12904-016-0080-0.

Singh Ospina N, Phillips KA, Rodriguez-Gutierrez R, Castaneda-Guarderas A, Gionfriddo MR, Branda ME, Montori VM. Eliciting the Patient's Agenda- Secondary Analysis of Recorded Clinical Encounters. J Gen Intern Med. 2019 Jan;34(1):36-40. doi: 10.1007/s11606-018-4540-5. Epub 2018 Jul 2. PMID: 29968051; PMCID: PMC6318197.

Sloterdijk, P. (2013). *You Must Change Your Life: On Anthropotechnics* (W. Hoban, Trans.). Polity Press.

Stadnitski T. Measuring fractality. Front Physiol. 2012 May 7;3:127. doi: 10.3389/fphys.2012.00127. PMID: 22586408; PMCID: PMC3345945.

Sun Simiao. "On the Sublime Sincerity of the Great Doctor." In Healing Virtue-Power: Medical Ethics and the Doctor's Dao, translated by Sabine Wilms. Portland, OR: Happy Goat Productions.

Tan, Richard. Acupuncture 1,2,3. January 1, 2007.

Tan, Richard. Dr. Tan's Strategy of Twelve Magical Points: Advanced Principles and Techniques. San Diego, California, 2003.

Tarver, D.E. The Art of War - Sun Tzu's Classic in Plain English With Sun Pin's : The Art of Warfare. iUniverseStar, April 19, 2002.

Tennant K, Long A, Toney-Butler TJ. Active Listening. [Updated 2023 Sep 13]. In: StatPearls [Internet]. Treasure Island (FL): StatPearls Publishing; 2024 Jan-. Available from: https://www.ncbi.nlm.nih.gov/books/NBK442015/

Thoreau, Henry David. *Walden; or, Life in the Woods*. Boston: Ticknor and Fields, 1854.

Unschuld, P. Huang Di Nei Jing Ling Shu: The Ancient Classic on Needle Therapy. University of California Press; First Edition, The Complete Chinese Text with an Annotated English Translation July 19, 2016.

Unschuld, P. Medicine in China: A History of Ideas, 25th Anniversary Edition, With a New Preface (Comparative Studies of Health Systems and Medical Care) (Volume 13) First Edition. University of California Press; First Edition, June 1, 2010.

Unschuld, P. Nan Jing: The Classic of Difficult Issues (Chinese Medical Classics). University of California Press; Second Edition, Revised July 19, 2016.

Unschuld, P. & Tessenow, H. Huang Di Nei Jing Su Wen: An Annotated Translation of Huang Di's Inner Classic – Basic Questions. University of California Press, 2011; First Edition, Volumes of the Huang Di Nei Jing Su Wen Project.

Vogel, Marcel. "Transformational Healing." marcelvogel.org, marcelvogel.org/transformational-healing.html. Accessed August 13, 2026.

West BJ. The Fractal Tapestry of Life: A Review of Fractal Physiology. Nonlinear Dynamics Psychol Life Sci. 2021 Jul;25(3):261-296. PMID: 34173731.

West BJ, Grigolini P, Kerick SE, Franaszczuk PJ, Mahmoodi K. Complexity Synchronization of Organ Networks. Entropy (Basel). 2023 Sep 28;25(10):1393. doi: 10.3390/e25101393. PMID: 37895514; PMCID: PMC10606256.

Wiseman, N., & Feng, Y. A Practical Dictionary of Chinese Medicine. Paradigm Publications, January 1, 2010.

Worsley, J.R. Five Element Constitutional Acupuncture, Vol. II: Traditional Diagnosis. The College of Traditional Acupuncture. First Edition, January 1, 1990.

Worsley, J.R. Five Element Constitutional Acupuncture, Vol. III: The Five Elements and the Officials. Redwing Book Co; First Edition, January 1, 1998.

Wright, Frank Lloyd. The Natural House. Horizon Press, 1954.

Xiang, L. Garden of Eloquence / Shuoyuan (Classics of Chinese Thought). University of Washington Press. January 16, 2022.

Young, Wei-Chieh. One Needle Therapy: Pain Syndromes. American Chinese Medical Cultural Center (First Edition, 2018).

Zhang, Jiebin. *Leijing* [The Classified Classic]. 1624. Volume 1, Life-Cultivation category. Chinese Text Project, ctext.org/wiki.pl?chapter=937085&if=en.

Zhang, C., et al. Foundation and Practice of Digital Traditional Chinese Medicine Platforms in Enhanced Recovery After Surgery. Future Integrative Medicine 2025 vol. 4(1) | 45–51 DOI: 10.14218/FIM.2025.00011

Zhāng Zhòngjǐng. *Shāng Hán Lùn* [On Cold Damage]. Translated by Craig Mitchell, Féng Yè, and Nigel Wiseman. Paradigm Publications, 1999.

Zhu SP, Luo L, Zhang L, Shen SX, Ren XX, Guo MW, Yang JM, Shen XY, Xu YS, Ji B, Zhu J, Li XH, Zhang LF. Acupuncture De-qi: From Characterization to Underlying Mechanism. Evid Based Complement Alternat Med. 2013;2013:518784. doi: 10.1155/2013/518784. Epub 2013 Sep 8. PMID: 24194782; PMCID: PMC3781993.

www.ingramcontent.com/pod-product-compliance
Lightning Source LLC
LaVergne TN
LVHW010715061126
851857LV00014B/1197